WALK
THE
LYME

WALK
THE
LYME

FROM KNOCKING ON DEATH'S DOOR TO
BUILDING A MULTIMILLION-DOLLAR BUSINESS

TAYLOR NELSON

LIONCREST
PUBLISHING

WALK THE LYME

*From Knocking on Death's Door to Building
a Multimillion-Dollar Business*

ISBN   978-1-5445-3856-3 *Hardcover*

        978-1-5445-3857-0 *Paperback*

        978-1-5445-3858-7 *Ebook*

CONTENTS

DISCLAIMER

specialist regarding the suggestions and recommendations made in this book.

Except as specifically stated in this book, neither the author nor publisher, nor any authors, contributors, or other representatives, will be liable for damages arising out of or in connection with the use of this book. This is a comprehensive limitation of liability that applies to all damages of any kind, including (without limitation) compensatory damages; direct, indirect, or consequential damages; loss of data, income, or profit; loss of or damage to property; and claims of third parties.

You understand that this book is not intended as a substitute for consultation with a licensed healthcare practitioner, such as your physician. Before you begin any healthcare program, or change your lifestyle in any way, you will consult your physician or another licensed healthcare practitioner to ensure that you are in good health and that the examples contained in this book will not harm you.

This book provides content related to physical and/or mental health issues. As such, use of this book implies your acceptance of this disclaimer.

AUTHOR'S NOTE

Some names in this book have been changed.

To Cody Parkin,
for always being a true friend to me
even in the hardest of times.

Lyme is isolating, and a lot of people
weren't there for me, but you always were.

From introducing me to the solar industry
before Lyme to letting me sleep on the floor
in your room when I got started to giving me
a hug in the car after an emotional collapse,
your friendship has been invaluable.

To Trey Pruitt,
for being a true friend and coming along
this ride of life with me for many years.
Your friendship never wavered, and your view
of me never changed, whether I was
kicking ass in life or I wasn't.

To everyone else who stuck around
even when I was at my worst.

FOREWORD

WHAT DO YOU BELIEVE?

Do you believe in God? Do you believe in fate? Do you believe everything happens for a reason? Do you believe that everything is random and sometimes bad things happen to good people? Do you believe that you have the power to change your destiny or path? Do you believe that life just keeps trying to keep you down?

I believe that bad things happen to almost everyone.

I believe that some things that happen to people are worse than other things. For instance, I lost my son to suicide when he was fourteen. For many families in similar situations, things never get better after that point. Others persevere and they find a way to move forward.

I met TJ Nelson about a year and a half after my son died. He wanted someone to coach him as a CEO, which happens to be what I do. His company, Direct Solar, is a hard-core, knocking-on-doors business. He faced a constant need to push, motivate, manage, and push again on his people to go out and knock on doors for five or six hours at a time to find leads that they would then go on to sell.

It's a tough business—not because it's hard to do, but because most people don't have the stamina or personal motivation to do the work, even though they can easily make $10,000–$20,000 a month just by being consistent. As the CEO/sales manager, TJ was constantly out knocking. He outsold all of his salespeople. He worked harder, plus he spent hours and days with his team to help make them better.

"And by the way, I should tell you, I have Lyme disease." This came out in our first conversation. I had no idea what Lyme disease was and how debilitating it actually can be. Through TJ, I soon learned.

Over the last couple of years, I have watched him go through so many different treatments, from stem cell injections in Mexico (which he turned me on to) to stinging himself with bees (which I opted not to do).

I spoke to him at low points and at times when he had hope. The one thing that has always been consistent with TJ is that no matter how much pain he was in, when he showed up for work, he showed up not just to play but to win! He may have had to down a cocktail of medications to be able to make it to a sales meeting, but he made it every time.

Even though he has seen dark times, TJ has never given up as he has learned to appreciate the little things in life and has battled both to build his business and to dominate his disease.

TJ is a hero, someone who I admire greatly. This is his story. I hope it inspires you as much as he inspires me.

Jason Reid
Partner, CEO Coaching International

Success is as dangerous as failure.

Hope is as hollow as fear.

What does it mean that success is
as dangerous as failure?

Whether you go up the ladder or down it,
your position is shaky.

When you stand with your two feet on the ground,
you will always keep your balance.

—TAO TE CHING

INTRODUCTION

I WAS DIAGNOSED WITH LYME DISEASE IN FEBRUARY 2017.

Since then, I have fought, accepted, and largely overcome the effects of Lyme. It has been brutal. I've run a marathon, beaten certain addictions and drugs, watched my parents get divorced, lost my real brother, lost my soul brother. Nothing compares to this.

Nothing in my life has been as hard as Lyme disease.

You're reading this book because you have Lyme or you care about someone who does. If your experience has been anything like mine, you feel misunderstood, isolated, lonely, and restricted. You can't do many of the things you used to do: traveling, dating, going out, doing physical activities, performing demanding work. The scope of your life has been sharply reduced.

You live in an internal, invisible prison. Many people suffering from Lyme look good on the outside. Most of the time when I had it, I looked great even though I felt horrible. Because of that, many people who don't have Lyme don't take it seriously. Neither doctors nor family nor friends believe Lyme is as real or as challenging as it is. They think we're pretending. Or we can cure it with mindset. Or it really isn't that bad.

Sometimes I looked awesome, but I felt terrible. I felt like I was running a marathon every hour of every day. A marathon asks you to give everything you have for four hours. Lyme asks you to give everything you have, every day, for years, to do the simplest of tasks.

Lyme takes different forms. It can mess up your joints and be present primarily in your body. It can mess up your head, creating confusion and memory loss. It can put you in a wheelchair.

Lyme can kill you, but it probably won't. It will just make you wish you were dead. Lyme kills you on the inside, but you're still alive on the outside.

I wished I was dead more than once. I decided to kill myself more than once.

Clearly, I didn't do that. Why not?

About eighteen months into my Lyme journey, I understood that as bad as I had it, many people had it much, much worse. I realized that I really wanted to help those people. I also realized that I couldn't do that until I helped myself. I can't fill another person's cup when my cup is empty and has a big hole in the bottom.

If you are suffering from Lyme, I want to help you. I wrote this book to help you. You who are suffering with Lyme disease, I see you! I understand you! I get you! I know what you are going through.

My goal in my journey was to to find the highest leverage points for healing and to get results without hurting myself. As you will read, I tried *everything*. I was a human guinea pig. I went up and down the physical and emotional roller coaster again and again.

It sucked.

I also wrote this book because I want the world to understand how much Lyme disease sucks. More and more people are getting it, but it's still very poorly understood. If someone has cancer, which is horrible, everyone understands what that means. We even understand if it's a really bad cancer or a not-so-bad cancer. We have some sense of how to help people with cancer.

In my experience, that cultural understanding and empathy doesn't exist with Lyme.

You'll find two parts to the book. The body of the book is simply my story: what I did, how I felt, what I went through, how Lyme affected my life, my ups and downs. Everyone's story is unique, but perhaps you'll see some of your own experiences in mine. If you do, I insist on this: you must also see that I have improved dramatically!

At the back of the book I have listed all of the supplements and medications I have taken and my experience with them. This is the second part. I am not endorsing any of these treatments for anyone else. I am only sharing my experience with them. You may learn about treatments or medications in this book that you would like to try yourself. What worked for me may not work for you. But I do want you to know about what I tried, so you have information about what you might try.

Of course, I'm no doctor and I'm not recommending anything in particular, nor am I liable for anything that happens if you do something you learned about here. I'm simply sharing my experience, so you may benefit from it.

Lyme is not a death sentence. Lyme is not a life sentence. You can manage it and live with it. You can improve slowly over time. It's important that you learn that from this book. It won't be easy, but you can do it.

Lyme sucks. Lack of awareness about the suffering Lyme creates also sucks. I hope my story, and what I've learned, make both those things suck a little bit less for you.

For a long time, my goal was to make it to the peak and back in one piece. I told myself I have to endure and stay the course. I have to win this battle to be an example to everyone else that they can win the battle too. I can't give up. And when I complete my climb, I can't wait to give back to you who are climbing the mountain, who may be running out of supplies, who might be losing the mental war halfway up, or who are just getting too cold from the isolation. That thought gave me a reason to continue. My journey goes on, and I hope it helps you.

CHAPTER

1

"Denial can be confusing because it resembles sleeping. We're not really aware we're doing it until we're done doing it."

"THERE HE IS!"

I lay completely naked in a bath that had gone cold, so tired I had been unable to get up for hours.

"What was that?" I had my friend Matt on speakerphone. He heard the shout too.

I sat up and turned to look out my sliding glass door. My neck was so stiff I couldn't fully rotate it. That's when I saw the four policemen staring at me. I felt nothing—no alarm, no curiosity, no fear, no surprise. I just registered a visual of what was occurring. Clearly, I was out of it.

"Oh, just the San Diego police that have closed in on me. I should probably see what they want," I said to Matt.

"Say what?!"

I hung up on him.

Standing up felt like deadlifting five hundred pounds. Slowly, I stepped out of the bath and wrapped a towel around my waist. My phone buzzed—Matt calling back. I ignored him and walked to the sliding glass window to let the cops in. They were laser-beam focused on me, watching my every move, as I shuffled toward them, leaving a trail of water on the fake hardwood floor.

I unlocked the sliding door, and four cops barged in.

"Take a seat," one of them said. I sat on the edge of my mattress as eight eyes drilled into me.

Still, I felt nothing.

Three of them relaxed a bit as their leader spoke to me. His eyes skimmed my body. "Why are your feet purple?"

I looked down. My feet were an entirely blueish-purple that resembled a fresh bruise about to form.

"Oh, I don't know," I said, waving my hand dismissively. But I did wonder, *Why the hell are my feet purple? How did I not notice that before?*

"What do you mean?"

"Well, I have Lyme, so I get weird symptoms."

He raised his eyebrows as he stared at my feet. "Interesting," he said slowly. "Does that make you feel bad? How are you right now?"

"I'm fine. How are you?" I replied, as if this was a normal conversation.

"Are you sure?"

"Of course. I'm good." The gravity of having policemen in my room still hadn't really registered with my broken brain.

"OK...and you don't have any thoughts of hurting yourself?" He peered into my eyes.

"No, not at all."

"Can you explain this?" The officer turned his phone around to show me a screenshot of a text I had sent out that morning to a handful of people—and I had completely forgotten about it after I got in the bath. The image was a Google Maps shot of San Diego's Coronado Bridge and a text from me reading, "I've had enough. I can't take it anymore."

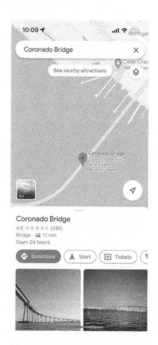

"Ohhhh. I know why you're here now."

"All right," he said. "I have to put these handcuffs on you. You aren't being arrested; you are only being detained. Do you understand?"

"Let me put my clothes on."

"We'll assist you with that." He seemed very at ease ordering me around.

Shit, I have to get naked in front of these guys?

It wasn't the most comfortable moment of my life, but I understood why they were doing it. They didn't want me to close the closet door and off myself while I still had the chance. They had to take every precaution to ensure I didn't do anything crazy.

I stood up and dropped the towel. Butt naked, I walked past them and into my closet to get my clothes. As I was picking out what to wear, the main guy snapped at me to "just grab something. It doesn't really matter."

I don't know why I'm trying to select an outfit. Who knows where I am going?

For some reason I wanted the colors to match up nicely, as if I were going out with friends. It's weird how you can act when your brain is broken.

When I was dressed, shit got real. "Hands behind your back."

They put the handcuffs on so tight they cut into my wrists. I'd never been arrested or detained before, so this was a new experience for me.

Two officers led while the other two flanked me. We stepped out to the street and waited for traffic to cross to their car, parked in the median turn lane. Part of me didn't care that I was being led away from my home. Another part was annoyed. But I also felt so alone, sick, and messed up that having the police bust in almost gave me a feeling of relevance. *Hey, I'm important enough for four people to grab me and escort me to a police car.*

I wonder if any neighbors are going to see this, I thought, but I had never talked to and didn't know any of them, so it didn't matter. *At least my roommate isn't here to experience all this.*

They put me in the back seat. Two of the cops sat up front; the others left in another car.

As we drove, I was still out of it—no idea where we were going. The lead cop piped up, "Where are you from?"

"Utah."

"Interesting."

"What do you mean?"

"Did you see my name tag?"

"Yeah, it says J. S."

"My name is Joseph Smith." He turned to meet my eyes before facing forward again. Then he laughed. I let out a little laugh myself. I could tell he used that line with everyone from Utah he encountered. Joseph Smith was the founder of Mormonism, and people seem to think everyone from Utah is a Mormon.

By this point in my life, I was completely numb. Nothing mattered. But in that moment, fate hit me. It hit me like the fatigue train that ran me over every morning when I tried to wake up.

As I hunkered down in that back seat I thought, *OK, I admit...I'm fucked up.* The heavier the truth, the harder it is to swallow. It took being placed in the back of a squad car for me to acknowledge it.

Utah. It was time to go home. It was time to get help.

CHAPTER
2

"Pride...limits or stops progression. The proud are not easily taught. They won't change their minds to accept truths, because to do so implies they have been wrong."

—EZRA TAFT BENSON

"THEY ARE GOING TO KEEP ME HERE FOR THREE DAYS?" I asked Officer Smith as he helped me out of the back seat. He and his partner walked me into a creepy psychiatric hospital that blended prison and medical aesthetics.

"Yeah. Per protocol, you have to stay here to make sure you are safe and not a risk to yourself."

Shit. I have zero supplements, no medications...nothing on me that I HAVE to take every day to be just above the brink of collapse. If I'm stuck here, I'm screwed.

I knew I had to pull it together and appear completely normal. If I was going to leave the hospital in less than three days, I had to figure out how to bend the rules with the people who ran the joint.

* * *

My life was unrecognizable the day the San Diego police came and took me away. I was doing things to try to regain my health that I would have told you were insane before they became a regular part of my life.

Maybe if you are reading this and have Lyme, you are afflicted mostly by joint pain and malaise. I don't have joint pain that bad. I have body soreness, tightness, pain, psychological issues, brain fog, inability to think, and worst of all, relentless fatigue. Fatigue so bad it hurts. This fatigue is like waking up, seeing that your phone is at 15 percent battery, and trying to get through the whole day on that charge. On top of that, the glass is cracked and the phone is damaged, making it glitch half the time you try to perform a function. That was all you'd have to work with—15 percent of who you know you could be.

I also have insomnia, and insomnia from Lyme is the most unreal form that exists.

I would wake up almost every night between 3:00 and 4:00 a.m. and be wide awake. Sometimes I was sweating. Sometimes I was cold. I'd get up and try to take chamomile extract or valerian root, hoping I could fall back asleep. It was torture trying and failing to fall asleep every night.

Do you know how hard it is to do anything with people when you feel tired out of your mind?

A few times, I had to do a coffee enema to be able to function that day—as odd as that sounds. Just the way a person drinks coffee to get going, I was doing a coffee enema to be able to drag myself through a social event.

For a while in San Diego, I strengthened my knuckles every day by punching a brick wall. I lifted a kettlebell by biting onto a T-shirt tied to it to strengthen my jaw. I would try to instigate fights because I secretly wanted someone to kill me. During that time, I learned how some people hit that point of no return. They don't care anymore; they are so dead inside it just...doesn't...matter.

I never actually got in a fight during this period because most people really don't want to fight. Only the folks who truly don't give a shit do. And the individuals I dared to throw down with probably looked in my eyes and saw I had nothing to lose. They knew to move on. I would even tell people, "If my blood gets on you, you will be infected with four diseases that will kill you." That sure amped up the craziness factor that warned them away. Of course, my blood wouldn't hurt them. But they didn't know that.

Until the cops got me out of the bathtub after I sent a suicide text, I had not understood how some people did stupid stuff that alters their lives forever. But now I know that when you're that sick—that fucked up—you just don't care anymore.

* * *

The officers, still flanking me, brought me to the front desk to check in. I explained who I was and why I was there. The girl at the front desk looked at me and sort of smiled. It wasn't a real smile, like someone feeling friendly toward you. I could see in her eyes that she saw me as a crazy person. I was more of an object than a human being, a thing you need to be careful of.

"Do you have any food? I haven't eaten all day."

"Yeah," the disinterested girl said. "We can get you a peanut butter sandwich and a carton of milk."

"I can't eat gluten or dairy."

"Umm...I don't think we have anything else." She shrugged. Clearly, she would prefer to be anywhere but here.

I won't be able to eat anything here either. Also, why the hell do places like this feed junk to people with psychiatric issues? Don't they know the role that food plays in mental health?

The cops placed me in a room and closed the door. Soon another woman was admitted. She rocked back and forth. I thought she might be a meth addict. At this point, who the hell was I to judge? *Who knows how long I'm going to be here? I might as well start making friends.*

"What are you in here for?" I asked.

"I don't fucking know! Probably just some BULLSHIT! I haven't done anything, and here I am again, motherfuckers!"

She ranted on, and I quickly realized I should've kept to myself. Clearly, normal conversation wasn't possible. She didn't seem like she was going to try anything crazy, but I also knew that someone that lost can lose their empathy and not care if you want to continue a conversation. And I'd lost my ability to know what others are going through a few times myself. People like that can't tell how you are doing or if you're bored with the conversation. They are too consumed by their own inner hell to see outside themselves.

A man in a white coat opened the door. "Taylor?"

"That's me."

"OK, follow me."

I followed the guy I assumed to be a doctor into another room. He didn't introduce himself, just started asking questions. I believed I was coming off as completely normal. To prove this point, I even asked him some common questions that I use at the beginning of sales appointments to get people to open up.

At the peak of my career, only a year earlier in Dallas, I had been the top door-to-door salesperson in the country for SolarCity, the nation's largest residential solar company at the time. I thought I was unstoppable—I couldn't get taken down by anything. Maybe that was my type A personality talking, but it had served me well. I knew how to sell. I loved connecting with people. And I needed to get out of this place.

I let the doctor know that I wasn't really going to kill myself. Of course not! I just wasn't feeling good and had been expressing my frustration and pain. I had no plans to hurt myself.

Then I made a bold move.

"My friend is driving over from Las Vegas to help me. He'll get here later today."

"What's his name?"

"Matt."

"Do you mind if I call him?"

I wasn't expecting this. Matt had no idea what was happening to me and no plans to come to my rescue.

"Yeah, no problem," I said calmly. "I can grab his number out of my phone."

He wrote down Matt's number and got up to make the call in another room.

Matt and I had done sales together; we knew how to synergize to get what we wanted. Maybe he'd figure it out on the fly.

After a few minutes, the doctor returned. "He's already on his way, and since you appear to be mentally healthy and have someone coming to help you, it's safe for you to go home." He gave me a guarded smile.

Holy shit! Matt knew. If that hadn't worked, I would have perished here over the next three days. Sales skills and a little maneuvering save the day once again.

I took a cab home. On the way, I called my friend Trey in Salt Lake City to fill him in. He agreed with me—I should come to Utah.

As I waited at home in San Diego for Matt to arrive from Las Vegas (he was really on his way, understanding that I must be messed up since I just had a psychiatric hospital call him), everything I'd just been through slammed into me.

Damn. I just escaped a psychiatric hospital within three hours when I was supposed to stay there for three DAYS.

When you are in a dire situation and trying to survive, you can become very, very creative about finding a solution. The human brain is built for survival, but it's weird.

It will try to convince you to kill yourself.

It will let you lie around eating Cheetos, watching crappy reruns on TV while you destroy your life.

It will let you send a group text that almost gets you committed.

But it won't let you perish—or stay committed—when you know you are in serious trouble.

CHAPTER
3

"Your self-esteem isn't measured by how you act and behave when things are going good. Your self-esteem is measured by how you treat yourself at your worst when all your vices and negativity come out."

—NATHANIEL BRANDEN, The Six Pillars of Self-Esteem

"IT'S ALL ABOUT THE PULLBACK. EVERYTHING YOU DO, you have to ease the sales pressure. If someone feels like you are pressuring them, they'll dig their feet in and resist you. If you allow them to say no and make sure they see that you don't care if they sign up, they'll be more likely to sign up."

In late 2016 I stood on a table outside a hip restaurant in Dallas, preaching my sales wisdom to six sales reps. They gathered around and recorded every word I said. Selling rooftop solar systems was a part of my soul, but I was leaving this job. I felt like a piece of me was dying. So I let it all out. I didn't care about hoarding my wisdom anymore; I imparted it all to the sales reps staring up at me. They wanted to know, and I wanted to help them.

Oh...and I was high on LSD too.

I didn't know what was wrong with my life, but I had to figure it out.

When I first moved to Las Vegas from Utah, where I was born and raised, to begin selling solar in 2015, I was struggling. My bed was a blow-up mattress on the floor of my friend Cody's room in his apartment in Henderson. He loaned me his motorcycle to drive out to my sales territory in Summerlin, an area twenty minutes west of the Strip, to go knock on doors. This is where I learned I could sell.

Previously I had sold new and used cars in Utah. Not long after I got out of college, I bought a ticket to Thailand and traveled until I ran out of money. I was trying to follow in the footsteps of internet personalities who coached entrepreneurs to be "location independent" with online businesses, but it didn't work. I tried Thailand, Vietnam, and Colombia. Finally, one of them told me if I wanted to be successful, I should learn to sell. That's how I ended up in car sales. I did that for eight months. The first month I tied for number one in sales, and the whole time I was there I was in the top half of the dealer's salesmen. But I was itching for something different. Cody offered me the chance to sell solar systems door-to-door in Vegas, and I took it.

It was really, really hard. I was in debt, sleeping on my blow-up mattress on Cody's floor. The manager who originally hired me retracted the job offer when I was on the drive to Las Vegas, so I actually arrived without a job. I had to convince another manager to hire me instead. I wasn't exactly getting off on the right foot. To make things worse, I had terrible anxiety about knocking on people's doors—which, of course, was the job! Precisely because it was scary, I decided I had to master it.

The difficulty obsessed me—I wanted to be great at it.

I was working for SolarCity, the residential solar company Elon Musk's cousins founded. My job was to convince homeowners to buy our solar photovoltaic systems and install them on their roofs. These things cost tens of thousands of dollars but could add value to their homes. Back then, we did mostly power purchase agreements or leases, which allowed the homeowners to get the solar installed at no upfront cost and simply replace their electricity bill with a better one. Once the systems were installed, homeowners typically had to pay very little to their electric utility, saving them money right away. Every time I walked up to a door, I was super anxious. I didn't know if the complete stranger I was going to meet was going to be pissed off that I disturbed them, slam the door in my face, tell me to fuck off, or threaten me.

That happened a lot. But sometimes something different happened. Sometimes I spent several hours in their home, designing and pricing their system, going over paperwork, getting to know them. By the time it was over they might have invited me to their cousin's wedding (for real, stuff like that actually happened).

And I loved that. I loved making that connection, and of course, I made a commission on the sales. In fact, commissions were the only way I made any money at all. If I didn't sell, I didn't eat. Doing this work addicted me because it was so challenging. It forced me to directly confront my limiting beliefs every time

I knocked on a door. My sense of who I was, what I was capable of, and whether I believed in myself was put under pressure every day. My results were there in black and white to show who I was.

I knew I had something to prove. When I was a kid, my older brother Nathan was pretty mean to me. He bullied me, roughed me up a bit, and beat me up verbally. When I was sixteen and he was twenty-three, he contracted peritoneal cancer, which is extremely rare. Only one doctor in the Huntsman Cancer Institute had seen that form of cancer in someone older than one year of age. Nathan never had a chance.

I once had to help him into an ambulance headed for the cancer center because his surgical incisions were ripping open from the inside out. He yelled at me to blow his head off with a shotgun, the pain was so bad.

On the day he died, I received a phone call that he was near the end.

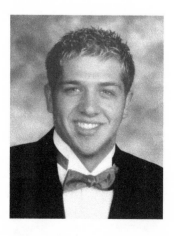

By the time I got to the hospital, he was already dead, bile dripping out of his mouth. Waiting for orderlies with a body bag to come and haul him off, I saw my father truly cry.

My brother died within a month of getting cancer, and it wrecked us all. He and my father were best friends, and he loved every second they spent together.

My family basically fell apart after that. I went from home to home for a while. I finished college at the University of Utah in 2012, where I had a full-ride scholarship because of my academic performance—and ended up living in low-income housing. I might have had a bachelor's degree in psychology, but I was poor, and it sucked. I didn't want to live in this poor-ass situation, where once somebody threatened me over my mountain bike, and another time I went into the laundry room and found a dead guy.

I was working, but I couldn't seem to make any money. This reality did not align with my self-image. I always saw myself as someone who could succeed at a really high level. I had to prove to myself that I could, and I had to prove it to the people who had doubted me. Before I got into solar sales, I had tried some other things. I started a website called Dominate Depression that tried to help people with courses, but it just limped along. I wanted to put my degree to use helping people, so I worked for the National Alliance on Mental Illness, but I found that working one-on-one with people drained me emotionally. I took on too much of their burdens.

I tried a couple of other random things to make money, including buying things on the internet and reselling them. I was all over the place trying to figure out what to do.

I developed a bit of a reputation among my friends and family as the guy who was always trying something new. I knew that people thought I wasn't going to succeed. When I worked for SolarCity I was determined to prove them wrong.

I worked seven days a week.

But after three months, the Las Vegas market shut down because the utility company stopped allowing homeowners to connect new solar systems to their power grid. The way residential solar power works, the utility has to pay or give credits to a homeowner for extra power they generate and feed back into the electrical grid. That is really important for making solar systems affordable for homeowners—they can actually offset their electricity bill so the solar payment, which is usually lower, replaces it.

It turned out that so much solar was being installed on rooftops around Las Vegas that the utility didn't want to lose any more money. They stopped approving new solar system connections. That killed our business. SolarCity gave the Vegas reps the opportunity to move to Dallas and sell there. I chose to go to Texas and from there, I rose to the top through sheer willpower and determination.

I loved selling solar in Texas. I became the top salesperson in my office. I kept upgrading my vision of what I wanted to achieve. First, I just wanted to pay off my debt. Then I wanted to pay my bills. Then I wanted to prove wrong the people who had doubted me. Then I wanted to donate a solar system to a school. I kept hitting my markers, which led to a drop in my motivation, so I had to set a new marker.

My sales manager would send me a screenshot showing how close I was to achieving some new high, and I'd hear a little voice in my head that said, "Whoa, can I really do that? I'm good, but not that good."

Then I'd pause and ask myself, "Hold up. Where did that voice come from? Did someone else put that in there from my past? Let's prove them wrong." And I'd go sell another deal. Sales was a way for me to continue to prove my own worth to myself.

Eventually, I decided I wanted to rise up to the level of becoming an icon in sales so I could show other people what is possible and give them permission to do the same. I wanted to help others have what I had.

One month—April 2016—I was the number one door-to-door salesman for SolarCity in the country, out of a couple thousand salespeople, according to a certain metric called a Power Ranking. That meant I was essentially the number one salesperson at the number one solar company in America. My average was twenty self-generated sales a month for three months in a row with a 90 percent pull-through ratio (meaning the people who signed contracts with me actually went to installation, rather than getting cold feet). One month I made $55,000. I averaged around $24,000 a month.

I was important.

I was on top of the world.

* * *

Now, it was all crumbling, and I didn't know why, which is how I ended up on LSD at a sales team dinner in Dallas in 2016. A friend had sent me LSD because I'd been depressed and couldn't figure out why. A little LSD might make me feel better. I was falling apart, and I thought it was because I was burnt out and needed to change out of the solar game—even though I loved my work.

Drugs had found their way into my life after my brother died. I tried a lot of things—marijuana, salvia, cough syrup, mushrooms. I did that for about a year when I was in high school. We were all fighting our own battles then. I needed another year to fully get off of drugs.

When I turned to drugs in a specific way like that—especially since I'd tried to abstain after being addicted when I was younger—it was a warning sign to me that something major (and likely bad) was happening in my life.

A year and a half into my solar journey and right after hitting massive numbers and setting records, I moved into my own apartment. Despite my outward success, I found myself feeling tired and depressed. I couldn't place my finger on why. I thought I was going insane, and anxiety ate away at me. That wasn't the way I normally felt. Something was wrong.

I developed bad brain fog and started to forget things. I've always been terrified of getting Alzheimer's, so this was a special kind of hell. I imagine once you realize you are losing your memory, the scariest part is knowing you are on the decline and that you will eventually not even know what is happening after you cross the point of no return. It would be like heading into a black hole knowing it was impossible to escape out the other side.

There is a saying that goes, "Wherever you go, there you are." Yeah—it took me a while to get my head around that one. Physically, I could pack up and leave in a heartbeat. Ever since I can remember, I have needed a way to escape or change course. Because of this instinct, I was really, really good at starting over in a new town, a new job. For years I tried to move somewhere else to fix my problems. This was my habit. I had moved seven times in the last few years to places I had never been before. Moving on seemed to work—or at least it provided a distraction for a little while.

When I look back on that behavior, I can understand it for what it was. I had—have, I suppose—a lot of abandonment issues. After all, my brother Nathan died when I was sixteen from a horrible cancer. My family fell apart, and my parents retreated into themselves. At one point I was living with my mom, and she usually wasn't around. She was never home, so my dad said I should live with him. Then he did the same thing. During college, I went from one home to another, and my best friend died. After I graduated, I finally landed in low-income housing, really the dumps, and hit a new low point.

I felt abandoned by everybody, at every level. I dealt with it by running away. Moving to another *city* didn't seem like such a bad idea now, since my running in the past had involved fleeing to different *countries*. In the years leading up to that point, I had lived in Thailand, Vietnam, and Colombia. As I mentioned, I was trying to do online business, and living in those countries was cheap. I bought a one-way ticket to Thailand to live cheaply and see if I could create a business just using my laptop. I moved to Vietnam because I had heard how cool it was. I tried to live in Colombia, but I got food poisoning twice during my various travels, which ruined my gut, and I couldn't make living in Colombia work. I wanted to get the "location-independent entrepreneur" thing to succeed, but I couldn't pull it off.

Now, struggling in Dallas and feeling burnt out, I looked for another change of scene, and a change of career too. I was going to leave solar sales and move to Austin. Maybe that would fix me.

But man, I felt like shit. When I tried to describe to people how I felt, they didn't really understand me. The best I could come up with was that I felt like I had a really bad flu. My whole body ached. I had pressure behind my eyes, and I had terrible brain fog. I couldn't focus, couldn't think well. I was totally exhausted. The difference was that most people had the flu for a few days. This went on day after day, week after week. (Later, I would tell people it felt like having COVID that didn't quit. A lot of people who had COVID could at least relate to that!)

I moved to Austin to try something new, convinced that I felt the way I did because of external reasons such as solar no longer being the right path and needing to make a change. But I was falling apart internally.

I was under a lot of emotional stress in Austin. I began to feel very anxious. I got depressed. I didn't realize it at the time, but at some point during my stay in Dallas, I must have picked up a tick and contracted Lyme. Like about 60 percent of Lyme sufferers, I don't remember ever being bitten. For a long time, I didn't know that what was actually happening to me was that I was slowly being destroyed by a pathogen. Instead, I thought that I must have lost my purpose, that I was depressed because I wasn't doing whatever it was that I was supposed to be doing.

By moving to Austin, I was looking for an external solution to an internal problem. When most people do that, their internal problem is psychological. But in my case my internal problem was physical. A pathogen was secretly ravaging my body and my life.

* * *

My heart broke as I left Dallas and what I had based my entire identity around—being good at selling solar. Little did I know, this wasn't the only thing that would collapse.

I wasn't all there. I didn't have energy. I didn't have the ability to focus. I didn't have my usual charisma, and I couldn't think straight. Just talking to my roommates gave me severe social anxiety. Something was wrong, but I still couldn't figure out what it was. Instead of looking deeper into it and slowing down to rest, I was determined to fix myself with willpower alone.

Willpower got me all my success. When I was knocking door-to-door in Texas, I underwent the most spiritual growth I ever had. Each of us carries psychological baggage—fears. Knocking on the doors of strangers and trying to convince them to spend tens of thousands of dollars forced me to face those fears. My brain was constantly telling me not to do exactly what I got up to do every day. Instead, I went out and visualized, on every street, "There's somebody here that's ready to go solar. They're there, and I'm going to find them."

I knocked on door after door, getting rejection after rejection. I got, no, no, no, no. I'd tell myself, "They're still out there. The deal's there. The deal's out there." Until finally I found them, and boom, I signed them up. It was kind of a "holy shit" moment to find success in the face of so much rejection. When I was starting out, I might knock three hundred doors before I signed a deal. Most skilled people knock about one hundred doors for every deal, on average. That's a lot of rejection.

I'd wake up and not want to go out to the field. I didn't want to do it, so I came up with various ways to harness my willpower. To force myself to confront all those internal doubts, all the external rejection. To will that deal into being. I would determine that I had some sort of internal limiting belief like, "I can't make $20,000 a month," and then I would set my willpower against that belief. I would go out to shatter that limiting belief, and I'd do it. Then I'd do it again.

That was a kind of spiritual growth.

Because I had learned to succeed this way, I wasn't about to admit that there was something actually wrong with me. I was determined to beat whatever was causing my depression and anxiety with willpower.

All it takes is mindset to win, I told myself again and again.

I got a job in a new field, working sales at an Austin tech startup. I was a wreck. I couldn't connect with my coworkers, and I was too tired to prospect and find new clients. I wanted to be back in Dallas doing what I did best—selling solar door-to-door. I'm still not sure if I was fired or if the owner and I both knew it wasn't a good fit, but after two weeks I was out of a job. I found myself living in a big house and a new city, unemployed and completely confused.

This was very threatening to my psyche, because like so many people, I defined myself by my work.

Although I didn't know it at the time, I was experiencing a cytokine storm, which is an immune system overreaction. My whole body had a nasty, achy "tight" feeling, like there was something in me that I wanted to rip out. I felt like shit, as if I were fighting off the flu, but different. I felt pressure in my head and behind my eyeballs. I was quick to anger. When I tried to wake up every day, it felt like I had run a marathon in my sleep. Everything was too much to handle. Just getting up to brush my teeth made me stressed. It was so hard.

With no work, no purpose, no direction, and a gnawing sense that I was heading toward failure and hopelessness that I tried to ignore, I fought to hold onto my identity. I went from being a near-celebrity in the solar sales world, with lots of friends and everyone wanting to be around me, to being lost and nobody wanting to come near.

When you are doing great, everyone wants to join in.

When you're not, it's a whole different story.

I have driven myself really, really hard my whole life because that's what I believe society demands of a man. The way I see the world, I have to be completely on top of my game. If I get sick, if my guard goes down for one second, I'm screwed. If I'm perceived as weak, my sales drop. My professional success collapses. Women who are dating me drop me and unleash their BS because they think I'm weak.

You may not agree with my worldview, and I don't believe that anymore myself, but that's how I saw things as I was flailing in Austin, feeling shittier and shittier.

When you are at your worst, even people who you thought were your good friends disappear. This is when you will learn how few people actually care. This was a hard truth to swallow.

Life was hitting me with all sorts of realities and truths I didn't want to accept. But you have to accept them.

* * *

A doctor in Austin named Jackman thought I was sick from Epstein-Barr virus (EBV), commonly called mononucleosis, which can lead to a lot of associated diseases. His prescription involved me ordering a lot of supplements from his personal store, including vitamins A and D, detox virus homeopathic remedy, lymphatic drainage homeopathic remedy, NAC (N-acetylcysteine), glutamine, lipoic acid plus, UltraVir-X, Bio-Immunozyme Forte, Se-Zyme Forte, Bio-FCTS, Betaine Plus HP, IAG, Bio-C Plus 1000, and Cytozyme-THY.

This would not be the last time someone tried to take advantage of me because I was sick. In fact, lots of people tried to take advantage of me. When you're sick, you'll do anything to feel better. This doctor, certain that all my problems came from EBV, insisted he could cure me with his natural supplements, so long as I kept buying them.

One morning I woke up with a weird red mark on my stomach, as if an alien inside me had made a curving red line on my abdomen.

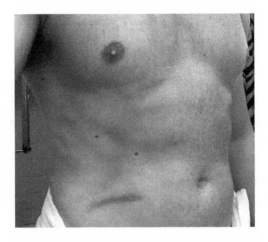

I had no clue what it was and didn't think too much of it. I took a picture of it and joked around about it with my roommates. My doctor had no idea what it was either. I heard a year or two later that he got sued for malpractice, so maybe he wasn't the person to ask.

Life got unhappier. Austin was not the place for me. I bailed out to Fort Worth, where I stayed with my good friend Cody, who lived there at that time. After a couple weeks there figuring out what I was going to do, I decided on San Diego, California.

I fit every single thing I owned in my Toyota Corolla *and* could still see out the back window. This was my life—minimalistic. About a quarter of the way to San Diego I started crying. I'm not talking about tears dripping down my face. No, I caved into an ugly cry, complete with body shaking and wailing. All the suppressed bullshit I couldn't let out in front of anyone else exploded out of me. I wasn't sure what I was doing, but there I was again, moving across the country to start over for the umpteenth time—driving away from my good friend Cody in Fort Worth.

I was abandoning Cody—just like I had been abandoned so many times.

I found a place to live and started my next gig. Although I am an extrovert by nature and hate being alone for extended periods of time (especially if I'm staring at a computer), I figured I would focus on internet marketing once again.

Each day I focused on building my business, but my health was slowly getting worse. Although I was holding onto reality the best I could, it kept slipping. I was scared, but instead of recognizing what was happening, I just kept believing I could overcome my health issues. *It's in the mind, TJ,* I would tell myself.

The symptoms were creeping up and intensifying so that I could see the incoming black hole: anxiety, depression, fatigue, confusion, brain fog, the inability to exercise. While I was overtaken with some symptoms that I couldn't ignore, others, like memory loss, were worsening imperceptibly. Given my fear of getting Alzheimer's, this was terrifying.

I didn't understand I was losing my memory until I had a conversation with a friend who said, "Oh yeah, remember this?" And I didn't. I didn't remember it at all.

"What the hell?" he said. "How could you not remember that?"

That started to happen again and again. Finally, he said, "Dude, I think you're losing your memory." That really freaked me out.

As I researched more about my symptoms, another rash appeared. It reminded me of the weird mark I'd gotten in Austin.

I looked it up and learned about Bartonella, aka cat-scratch fever. *What the hell is that? I don't remember a cat ever scratching me.*

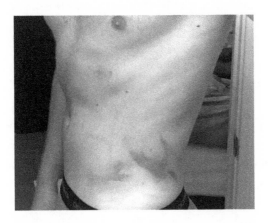

I started hitting up all the doctors in San Diego that could help me. Everyone wanted $450-plus for the initial consultation. They all had extremely long waiting periods too. I couldn't wait six months for a diagnosis. I had to find a way to figure out what the hell was happening.

I called one practitioner's office every single day until the front desk people and nurses all knew who I was and why I was calling. They seemed to appreciate my persistence as I hunted for a cancellation.

There's an indefinable quality about a person who calls every single day for help, with the determination of someone who is losing their life. The people on the other end started to take me seriously. My persistence created sympathy and made others want to help me. Only a person who is truly suffering would call every single damn day trying to get in. Only they would use every tactic possible to make that happen.

When I finally got an appointment, the guy I had been determined to see, Dr. Alex Whittaker, had no bedside manner. I felt like an animal in a factory being shuttled around and scrutinized like a science experiment.

I don't care if this doctor wants to yell at me during the entire appointment if he cures me.

The doctor went over random questions and areas of my life and health so we could look into them for answers. I described the scratch and showed him the picture. That got his attention. His bedside manner changed.

He touched my joints and asked if they were sensitive. He took a scanner and ran it over my knees, then said, "You have tendonitis in your knees." It was also apparent by the surprise on his face that what he was finding wasn't normal for my age. Dr. Whittaker asked me a few more questions, then drew a bunch of blood and ordered a ton of tests. Luckily, I still had health insurance from SolarCity, so I didn't have to pay the $2,000-plus price tag.

The results were eye-opening.

I tested positive for EBV (again), *Bartonella quintana, Bartonella henselae,* Lyme, Rocky Mountain spotted fever, and possibly mycoplasma.

My reaction to getting these results was, *What the shit is all that?!* I had never heard of most of these diseases and conditions.

When I looked up Rocky Mountain spotted fever, I read there was up to a 30 percent chance of death if left untreated. *This isn't good.*

I didn't even know what Lyme disease is. Lyme is a spirochete—a bacterium shaped like a corkscrew—that can change into three different forms. In other words, it's a conniving, tricky bastard.

The *Borrelia burgdorferi* bacterium is what people are referring to when they say "Lyme." Lyme has been around for a long time and has multiple strains, but Burgdorferi is the one messing everyone up.

Borrelia burgdorferi has a long DNA sequence and is complicated as hell. The spirochete gets deep into your body where it is hard to reach with antibiotics. It gets into your brain and joints, anywhere it can. It mimics a bunch of different diseases, too, so getting an accurate diagnosis is difficult.

Because of all this, people who struggle with Lyme for years can end up in wheelchairs or be completely destroyed by neurological problems. In that sense, the rapid progress of my Lyme disease was a lucky break. My symptoms got so bad, so fast, that I couldn't ignore them.

The doctor told me to take Plaquenil, a blood thinner that I forgot the name of, and an antibiotic. I was against antibiotics, so I never took what he prescribed me, and I never went back to his office.

My relationship with antibiotics over the coming years would be a complicated one. At this stage, I didn't want to take them because I had a broad distrust of doctors handing out pills and calling them cures. As I had struggled with depression, doctors told me, "Oh, just take this antidepressant," and prescribed a pill. None of those prescriptions worked for me. Eventually, I learned

I was deficient in vitamin D and magnesium. I changed my diet and relieved my symptoms. I didn't need antidepressants.

I had a belief that the medical industry gave everybody antibiotics for everything, and I felt that was a pretty messed-up approach. I thought doctors should try the natural route first, and that's what I was determined to do here. My experience with depression definitely colored how I approached the diagnosis I now had for tick-borne diseases.

My belief that antibiotics were bad might have been helpful for some people. If someone has a cold and is taking antibiotics when they don't really need them, that's not a good idea. But I learned the hard way that antibiotics are often very necessary to heal from Lyme.

Some doctors don't realize that 50 percent of their job is being a doctor, and the other 50 percent is being a salesperson. You have to sell the person on why they need to change their behaviors. Lyme is hard to treat because it is expensive, and there are long waiting lists to see the specialists. Dr. Whittaker definitely didn't understand the sales side of his job.

That appointment cost $890, but I didn't care—I was just grateful I had been able to see a doctor quickly. When you want to die every day from pain, waiting three months to see a doctor is unbearable and dangerous.

Funnily enough, looking back and knowing what I know now, Dr. Whittaker actually had tried to put me on a good regimen. But I had my beliefs, and I was sticking to them. I had used willpower to achieve so much in my life that I was determined I could use it with this problem too. Every day I had used willpower to defeat the negative voice in my head, to disprove my own limiting beliefs about what I could do in sales, so I thought, "OK, I'll just use my mind. I'll power through it. I'll take natural stuff and I'll beat it."

I was convinced that with willpower and strength of character, I had the tools to beat any diagnosis.

I found a different doctor, Dr. Casey, in Idaho, who didn't believe in antibiotics, either. He told me he had lots of experience with Lyme. After the initial consultation, he put me on supplements and powders and sent me a device called a ZYTO scan that plugged into my computer. When I put my hand on it, it supposedly sent biofeedback signals to him so he could remotely diagnose my situation and help me in real-time. He had been recommended to me by a woman I met who said he had helped her. Personal recommendations meant a lot to me. If he helped her, he might be able to help me. I was willing to give it a try.

I began his treatment, unaware that as I did so, all my dreams would begin to vanish, and I'd enter the pure nightmare hell of Lyme disease. Then I'd be left with just one dream, one wish, one desire in my life. To be healthy again.

CHAPTER
4

"You should take the approach that you're wrong. Your goal is to be less wrong."

—ELON MUSK

ONE OF THE SCARIEST PARTS OF LYME IS THAT IT CAN change *who you are*. That's because it burrows into your head, creating brain fog, anxiety, fear, confusion, impulsivity, memory loss, and a loss of self. That's the hardest part to experience, losing sight of yourself and feeling like you are someone else.

Every day I woke up in unbelievable pain. For hours I would lie there and tell myself, "You've got to get out of bed, you've got to get out of bed, you've got to get out of bed." My whole body hurt. I felt like I'd been run over by a car while I was asleep. I felt like I was in concrete. Everything, even getting out of bed, took so much energy. Outwardly, I looked fine, so people expected me to be fine.

What was going on inside my head was even worse. The whole world had a melancholy fade to it, as if it had no color. I couldn't find pleasure in anything. I could expect a whole day of feeling like this. And then another. And then another. A seemingly endless future of depression, anxiety, brain fog, pain, and feeling mentally handicapped.

Every day, my brain asked me, *If there's a 100 percent guarantee that the rest of your life will be like this, what's the point?* Because there was no point living that way.

Because I had no idea if or how or when I was going to get better, I had to create little carrots for myself, like a carrot on a stick to lead a donkey. I called them suicide carrots. I'd make a deal with myself. "All right," I'd say, "if I still feel this way at the end of the year, then I can kill myself."

That's how I got out of bed every day.

Two friends invited me to dinner in San Diego. By this point, I knew that many foods gave me really bad reactions. Lyme was making me sensitive to everything. Gluten, sugar, dairy, and anything processed caused bloating, pressure behind my eyes, and pain in my entire body—this would last for days.

But denial is a strong force in me. I was determined to continue to eat out, even though I often ate something I was sensitive to by mistake. If that happened, I had to deal with the pain and suffering afterward.

I'm a guy who loves to cold call, who loves to door knock and sell people. But lately my anxiety had been getting really bad. As I got ready to go out to the restaurant that evening I was beyond nervous, trying to fend off almost panic-attack-level anxiety.

I managed to get in the car, and while I drove, I rehearsed everything I would say at dinner, amping myself up not to be nervous. Instead of looking forward to dinner with my friends, I felt like I was about to address the nation on how to avoid a nuclear attack from a foreign country.

At the restaurant I was jittery, nervous, and analyzed every movement I made, every word I said—plus my friends' words. They couldn't tell that I was messed up inside. But I was certain that if I said or did the wrong thing I could screw up our friendships forever. On the way home I thought, *What in the actual hell? All I did was meet two friends for dinner, and I nearly had a panic attack. That's not normal, my man.*

Sales is funny because, on the one hand, you have to stay humble and know that you can always do better. On the other hand, when knocking doors, it benefits you to be totally convinced that you are the best solution for your client, that your product is amazing, and that you are God's gift to the planet.

The sales prospect will see your confidence, like your energy, and want to invite you into their home.

I used to be really good at that. Really good. Now I could barely converse with friends at dinner. My confidence had taken a huge hit, and I didn't understand why.

Our identity is based on a lot of factors that we are unaware of. We think we know who we are, but we simply string together a few facts about ourselves and say, "That's me." My identity was wrapped up in being healthy and strong. My identity was that I was smart and sharp. My identity was that I was a workhorse and a top producer. My identity was that I had energy and charisma. I could travel, go to conferences, and vibe with anybody. Now, I was losing all that.

My ability to understand books and solve problems was deteriorating. My earnings had dropped too. Not long before I was making $24,000 a month in sales commissions. Now, I began to refocus on running my site Dominate Depression, selling courses to help people get out of their depression when I was going into one of the most intense mental and physical battles of my life. I was scraping by on $2,000 a month from my online pursuits.

I was fighting to hold onto everything that was important to me. I was determined that I could beat Lyme with willpower, commitment, and energy. I told myself I was stronger than the disease was. Yet I was losing that battle. The truth of living with Lyme hadn't hit me full force, but it was going to. It continued to eat away at my sense of who I was and what I was capable of.

* * *

My anxiety and associated depression kept getting worse. I had to urinate and defecate before any social event. I thought the anxiety was externally created, and so I had to overcome it, just as I overcame so many other things. I joined an improv class to try to overcome my anxiety. Still, on class nights I had to arrive early and go to the toilet beforehand or make sure I did at home before leaving.

While I was in the class my heart would pound. The tension and craziness led to some wild performances, and I took heart knowing that some of the best entertainers have bad anxiety or stage fright, and that is *why* they do so well. But this was not healthy. I was moving toward a crippling condition.

The anxiety was relentless, just pounding and pounding on my brain. My brain was on fire all the time. *If this is what our life is going to be like forever,* it kept telling me, *just kill yourself.*

I continued to deny to myself that there was something seriously wrong with me that was outside of my control. Every now and then I went to the gym to exercise, but each time I hurt more and more. The hurt didn't feel like the typical pain you can get when you overdo it at the gym. When I lifted even light weights, a day or two later pressure formed behind my eyes; I would lose my appetite; I couldn't digest food; I would get insomnia and be completely wrecked for a good part of the week.

But I kept going. Going to the gym and feeling like shit became something I kept doing because I couldn't accept what was happening to me. I couldn't accept that I didn't have control. I'd look in the mirror and watch my muscles slowly decaying. My body was telling me I wasn't all that I thought I was. I couldn't control my destiny. I couldn't force my will to make all the pain and suffering go away.

It didn't matter that I had spent years building myself up; the universe could take my strength and body away from me whenever it wanted to. But I didn't want to accept that because I didn't want to see my body weaken and lose the work I'd put in and valued.

* * *

I got another referral to a doctor in Del Mar. She could get me in right away. That made me doubt that she knew what she was talking about. I figured she wasn't in demand. I now know that a shorter waiting list doesn't necessarily mean that.

My first visit was mostly paperwork, questionnaires (for what felt like the millionth time), and blood work. I returned for my results and sat with Dr. Krzyszinski. As I sat in her office, going over my symptoms and how I was feeling—the malaise overtaking me, the degradation in my health, the brain fog that made it hard to function—I asked her, "What is it looking like? Are you able to get me better?"

She looked at me, her face solemn yet controlled, like she was holding back the inevitable words that she had to say. I could see that she did not see me as just another number in the list of patients she had to get through that day. We were able to make a human connection—something I hadn't felt much of with my previous doctors. That kind of connection is incredibly important to me. I hungered for it, especially because I had dealt with so much abandonment. I cultivated it, too, and I used my skills in creating it in my sales career. So when I understood that this doctor got me, and she cared about me, I took her very seriously.

I've always had hope in life. I have *always* been able to fix my issues or get out of any tight situation. This time, based on Dr. Krzyszinski's reaction, I was afraid I was in over my head.

I could tell by her body language and hesitancy in answering that she didn't want to tell me the truth. People think that we communicate through what we say and the words we use. In reality, it's often what we don't say or our body language that truly communicates what we are thinking or feeling.

She wouldn't answer me, so I spoke up. "Lyme is permanent, isn't it? It isn't curable, and it is going to completely alter my life, potentially forever, and this is the way it is now."

She nodded, her eyes expressing true concern as she said, "Yes, it is manageable, but it doesn't go away."

At that moment I felt the horrible, weak, powerless sensation we feel when someone close to us dies. There is nothing you can do except take that body blow of grief. Except this time, it wasn't grief over someone else. Part of me was dead, and I needed to grieve *me*.

I broke down crying in her office. I couldn't help it. It just started coming out, almost as bad as the ugly cry I experienced on my move to San Diego. I cried like a little child who just needs a hug from his mother and to hear that everything will be OK, even though it won't. The life that I knew was over.

As the doctor watched me, I could tell this moment was hard for her. She might have been new to her practice and adjusting to not taking on the emotions and problems of her clients. Or maybe she actually cared.

Dr. Krzyszinski prescribed antibiotics and natural treatments, but I refused them and left. I couldn't bring myself to accept those antibiotics because if I did, I would be accepting that I was really, truly sick. That I really, truly could not beat this thing with willpower and character, which I relied on for so much in life. I wasn't ready to accept that. My denial was too strong.

I got to my car and drove aimlessly, not caring where I was going.

I felt worthless. Nobody would like me anymore. People had already left me. The less successful I was, the more they distanced themselves. I was convinced that if I was sick I would be messed up and tired at work. I wouldn't be able to produce. I wouldn't be able to deliver value for other people. And because I couldn't do that, they wouldn't like me and wouldn't want to be my friend.

Looking back now, I can see that I was not differentiating between good, true friends and friends who saw me as someone who could do something for them or get something for them—transactional friends. I thought those transactional friends were real. Because I was so hungry for human connection in my life, because I had been abandoned in so many ways, and because my brain was broken by Lyme, I leaned into those transactional friendships as if they were reliable. When I saw these people pull away from me as I got sick because they weren't truly invested in the friendship, that was a very painful kind of rejection.

If I am doomed to suffering, brain fog, and panic attacks just to go eat dinner with a friend, I might as well start getting rid of friends before they can get rid of me.

I texted my good friend Jeff that we "probably shouldn't be friends anymore." I had known Jeff for years. We met at an entrepreneur event in the Philippines and had remained in touch ever since. "I'm just not a good friend to be around." I don't know why I sent that to him specifically. I was in a self-destructive state and apparently my relationship with Jeff was the first thing I was going to destroy.

I drove until I got to a random beach, parked, and walked up a small hill. I sat in the dirt, arms draped on my knees. People below me surfed and played volleyball—things I couldn't do anymore. Everyone was having a blast. As I stared down at them, a prisoner peering into the outside world, knowing it wasn't for me, I was trapped behind bars, unable to do what everyone outside of those bars could.

Except there weren't any bars. I looked great on the outside. I looked healthy. But I was gone. My prison bars were inside my head and body. They were my life, invisible to the outside world and only visible to me.

As I sat there on that hill, I thought about all the things I couldn't do anymore.

I can't donate blood.

I can't exercise.

I can't travel.

I can't go to conferences.

I can't brush my teeth without being exhausted.

I can't surf.

I can't do yoga.

I can't hang out with a bunch of friends.

I can't go to parties.

I can't stay up late.

I can't drink alcohol.

I can't work.

I can't...do anything anymore.

I sobbed on that hill until my phone rang.

"Yo, what's going on, man?" Jeff said.

"Nothing." I knew Jeff could hear I had been crying. He didn't normally accept feelings of despair as valid responses, but this time he asked, "Are you all right?"

"I have Lyme disease, bro. I'm fucked."

"I knew something was wrong. People don't just randomly throw away a long-lasting friendship for no reason."

He was right. No one else would throw away a friendship like ours.

When you are hurting that badly, you need another person to hear you out. You need to feel seen. That day, Jeff did that for me. You know someone is a true friend when you can be a totally crazy bastard toward them, and they know that isn't you. They will call you up because you have given them a warning sign that everything isn't OK. They won't abandon you. They will hear you out and walk alongside you as you get better. I was blessed by Jeff's friendship. He had taken the time to call me and hear me. I needed that.

The phone call with Jeff helped me to see reality a bit more clearly. We could remain friends. Even though I felt a little better, I sat on the hill and stared out into the abyss of the ocean for a while. I wasn't used to being *this* alone. As an extrovert, I always wanted to be around people. I was one of those wild people who *enjoyed* knocking doors. Now here I was alone.

Being alone would become a common theme on my Lyme journey. I had been running away from myself for a lot of my life. My whole life had been some form of running, chasing after something. If I just get good grades I can get into college, if I just finish college I won't be poor, if I just move to this country or this city I'll find success, and people will like me. If I just prove myself my family will love me. If I just work hard enough, if I just make a big enough mark on the world, I will fill the hole in my heart that was left when my brother died, when my best friend died, when my family fell apart.

This time, I was sick and could no longer run. All my dark parts were catching up to me. They were standing over me, staring me right in the eyes while I was down.

I drove home, unsure what I was going to do. I was lost. I had nothing. But I also knew I had overcome challenges before. Whatever the problem, in my worldview the solution was to take action. Some kind of action.

* * *

I decided to join a Lyme support group in San Diego. I figured I could get around similar people I could relate to.

Maybe I can even make some friends who understand everything I've been doing to get better.

I also joined a San Diego conscious community group on Facebook. These people were into meditation, eating healthy, and being environmentally conscious. I started posting about what was going on with me in both of the groups. Soon, a person from the conscious community reached out to me. He invited me to his house, and we chilled on his balcony. He began preaching about everything I already knew about Lyme. He said he just wanted to help me and that he was a "coach."

"How much money," he asked, "do you have in your bank account?"

That's an odd question.

He started a sales sequence on me.

Ohhhhh, that's what this is.

His coaching cost $5,000 a month.

I soon made my excuses and left. Later I shot him a text, giving him sales pointers and letting him know that his bait and switch didn't work.

He sent back a long text, saying, "I am in integrity with God. Only God can judge me."

He was the first of many people I encountered who wanted me to pay them insane amounts of money to be my "coach." After that, I isolated myself more. My brain fog was making it harder and harder to judge people and know their true intentions. I didn't trust myself to know who was or wasn't trying to screw me over in my vulnerable state.

My other problem was that I loved to work. The statement "You work too much" assumes that the work is unenjoyable or not a good way to spend time. When you are passionate about what you are doing, instead of watching movies on Netflix, you're creating your own movie in real-time. You're doing what you love.

Some of us are simply wired differently. We each have a different purpose and might get more satisfaction from rest, quiet, beaches, relaxing. I love all those things, too, but only rarely and if I need it. Mostly, I love production and the challenge of making a business work.

Sure, people want lots of free time, but they want to use their time in fulfilling ways. Nobody is happy having a shitload of free time, doing nothing. I don't personally know anyone that is truly happy after watching Netflix all day, confronted by three empty ice cream cartons.

When people have questioned my commitment to work, the conversations have gone something like this:

"You work too much."

"What else would I be doing?"

"Watching a TV series, movies, going out and exploring."

"I hear you. Why do you do those things?"

"Because they are fun and enjoyable."

"I love my work, and it's fun and enjoyable, so I'm basically doing the equivalent of those things but all day long."

"…"

Obviously, I loved to work and found it very hard to not be working. I am a type A personality. I wanted to be a producer. Yet now, faced with a Lyme diagnosis, unable to do what I love to do, increasingly ill, and isolated, I had only two events to look forward to in my life: a Lyme support group on Saturday and an improv class on Tuesday evening.

I had joined the Lyme group thinking I'd meet some people who would understand me and learn some things that could help me get better. Before the support group meeting, I got myself all fired up, and I arrived full of enthusiasm. I had done a bit of Lyme research, reading stories about various treatments different people had tried, and gained some optimism that I'd find a way back to health.

One person was in a wheelchair. Everyone wore a green shirt to represent Lyme, but no one was smiling. I took my position in the circle. When it was my turn to speak, I explained that I'd just found out I had Lyme, people didn't believe I was as sick as I felt, and they didn't know what Lyme was, but I was looking forward to beating it and learning how to win.

When I was done, a blonde woman in her late thirties who looked healthy on the outside just like me, with the facial expression of not giving a shit anymore, said, "I've had Lyme for eight years. You're fucked. Nobody believes me either. My own brother doesn't believe that I am as sick as I am. Nothing has really worked for me."

Oh, shit. That's not what I want to hear.

Everyone else shared similar experiences. They were so beaten down. Lyme had torn up the joints of the woman in the wheelchair so badly that she couldn't really walk anymore.

No way...What the hell is going on?

My shoulders sagged as I left, my heart broke. I had gone in with optimism, looking to find ways to win, but I left destroyed and hopeless.

That experience became a common one with Lyme and me. Time and again, I met someone, learned something, heard about a new treatment—something happened to get my hopes up. Time and again, things didn't go as I had hoped. I didn't get better. Often, I felt worse. After a while, I learned not to get my hopes up, as I was likely to fall back down into sickness again—no matter what I did.

Goddammit. What am I up against?

* * *

On days I couldn't get out of bed, or it was too painful for me to move, I opened up liquid rhodiola rosea capsules and rubbed them under my tongue, but they didn't help.

Dr. Casey, in Idaho, recommended new supplements from Xymogen. He stated that serrapeptase is the number one supplement I should be taking, and we would monitor my CD57 results, which is a marker of the immune system. The results supposedly measure how well you are doing with Lyme. A lower number means you are not doing well. I took Takuna for two weeks, then Cumanda for two weeks, cycling back and forth. I took Sida acuta for Babesia, stevia drops for Lyme, and Banderol for Lyme and coinfections in general (which I still take). I was on Colostrum, glutathione, para-gard, digestive enzymes, MegaSporeBiotic, OptiCleanse GHI, Astaxanthin, CoQ10, Colloidal Silver spray, etc.

I was spending lots of money. None of it was working.

I didn't know why I trusted this random doctor I'd never met in person more than the other doctors. But I did. Probably because, like me, he didn't think I should take antibiotics. He claimed that herbs alone were more powerful than medications. "They are all you need," he said.

Except I kept getting worse. More anxious than ever, I isolated myself more. I become more and more messed up. New markings appeared on my body all the time. Dr. Casey believed the markings that bubbled up were Babesia- and Bartonella-related.

Depending on the mark, I took Cumanda for Bartonella or Sida acuta for Babesia. I also took Banderol for Lyme in general.

* * *

I started researching Lyme treatments. I concluded that an infrared sauna would be a good addition to my regimen—it would help me detox as I killed off pathogens, which I hoped I was doing. My friend Jeff let me rent his infrared sauna. I put it in the rental house I was in even though my roommate hated it. Of course, he wanted to put a couch where the sauna went, but I knew the sauna was necessary. When you are dealing with what feels like life-or-death, you start doing shit and not caring about people's approval. The sauna wasn't a want. It was a need.

At this point I was simply coping, existing, randomly playing a stupid little game off the app store on my phone or watching YouTube interviews with Joe Rogan. I got on Tinder or other dating apps and tried different combinations of phrases to get girls to come over to me since I didn't have the energy to go on dates. That made me feel like I was productive, but I wasn't thriving.

Because I didn't feel like I had unconditional love, I believed I had to earn love and acceptance. I did that by producing—by working hard, making money, helping people. If I couldn't do that, who would want to be around me? Who would care for me?

Given that mindset, it was hard for me to focus on being alive and trying to meet all my basic needs. Yet for eight months in 2017, I lived a life in San Diego that increasingly did just that. On a typical day, I might take hours to get out of bed, fighting my mind and my body to get up and get going. When I finally did, I'd eat a little breakfast. My diet was already pretty restricted from the stomach illness I'd had when I lived abroad. I ate a lot of frozen hash brown potatoes, which seemed to work OK for me, but I got pretty tired of them. Then maybe I'd take a short walk. Once I had the infrared sauna, I'd sit in there for half an hour. Then I'd take a detox bath of Epsom salts, baking soda, and essential oils, sometimes for hours. I'd lie in the bath, unable to get up.

When I finally got out of there, I'd try to do a little work or just watch YouTube videos to take my mind off how I was feeling. If I didn't have an obligation to get me out of the house I could easily fall into a semi-vegetative state.

I fell off the treatment wagon here and there. Every now and then, I would numb out and eat a bunch of weird food I shouldn't eat. I'd take some drugs, or watch random YouTube videos or porn. I was trying to hide and not deal with how I felt about everything. I kept trying to avoid my feelings and even physical sensations but would slip up and do self-damaging things. Those types of destructive behaviors are an indicator light. They let you know something is wrong and needs to be examined. They alert you to a symptom. When you are going through a challenge as rough as Lyme, you have to learn to love every part of yourself, even the worst vices and coping mechanisms—because they will emerge.

I wasn't there yet.

Sometimes I was so frustrated. I'd think, "I'm losing my life! I'm wasting away here." That was usually when I did something weird and fell off the wagon. Otherwise, every day felt like purgatory, just waiting for something to change, for this awful feeling to be over. I had to accept that I was sick and couldn't really live my life. For a couple of years, when I turned twenty-six and then twenty-seven, I didn't even want to count the birthdays. I didn't feel like I could count those lost years.

One day in 2017 I hit a moment of clarity and sat down and wrote a poem to explain my internal prison of suffering. I wanted the cycles to end. The poem was my way out...but I knew it wouldn't change anything.

This Time Will Be Different

Here I try to admit

That this is it

That this time is different

Well, it is, but it isn't

I've tried to run and deny

Hide behind a wall of innocent lies

They say God is always watching and always sees

But in reality, that person is actually me

Before, I'd beat myself up and feel down

I'd fill my skull with the sludge of self-pity and drown

I thought this time would be different

Well, it is, but it isn't

I'm compelled to make an elaborate plan

Then I laugh and know that that too will be damned

It can take one thousand times to have a lesson hit my core

There only is the present wave; there is no distant shore

I'm instantly forgiven, and I haven't gone mad

There actually is no good or bad

This is why this time feels different

Well, it is, but it isn't

This knowledge may be lost in five or seven days

Survival brain kicks in and has marvelous tricks and ways

Yet, I write this all in a loving and matter-of-fact tone

Fear is not the answer when I can get reality to speak to me alone

This regression is, in fact, mild

This part of me is to be loved like a lost and confused child

Once I let go of judgment and perfection

My higher resolve can breathe and take direction

I laugh as I realize that this time actually is different

I mean, it is, but it isn't

For I've tried to look outside to others, God, or religion

And forgotten to turn up my own inner voice, honor that, and listen

CHAPTER
5

"If opening your eyes, or getting out of bed, or holding a spoon, or combing your hair is the daunting Mount Everest you climb today, that is okay."

—CARMEN AMBROSIO

"YOU WILL NEVER TRULY BE GOOD ONSTAGE," THE INSTRUCtor said, "until you are comfortable and don't feel extremely nervous the whole time you are up there."

I am an adrenaline junkie. I have tried everything from skydiving with my own parachute to driving a bullet bike way too fast on the freeway. So it made a certain amount of sense that, as my anxiety ramped up, I decided to take stand-up and improv acting classes. I was determined to confront head-on the thing that I was most afraid of. I wasn't just going to confront it—I was going to become awesome in the face of it.

What the instructor meant was that I had to get on the stage and fail over and over and over. I had to deal with bad sets and jokes bombing until I truly gave zero fucks. Once I could get up and give zero fucks, that's when I would win.

Stand-up comedy was a true challenge. Of all the shit I've done, stand-up was the ultimate fear and rush. My anxiety amped me up, and I was so scared to practice in front of the class that I spent my time crafting jokes, studying punchline delivery, and practicing over and over to make sure I got it right.

Practicing stand-up comedy distracted me from my suicidal feelings, which grew more powerful every day. I reasoned that Rocky Mountain spotted fever might kill me anyway, since there was a 30 percent chance of death. I read that some of my coinfections could kill me too.

I used to wonder why old people never tried to hang on as long as possible. Some old people seemed more at peace with death than others. My grandfather, who suffered from colon cancer, used to tell me that he wanted to die. I didn't get it. Until Lyme.

I read that Lyme doesn't ever really kill people, although people with Lyme wish it did. I began to relate to the suicide stories of people who'd had Lyme. I looked up a story about a kid who isolated himself. After six months of Lyme, he committed suicide. That wasn't helpful. I was feeling worse and worse and worse and worse, so bad I wanted to die.

Maybe I'm on the decline to death. Maybe I won't have to commit suicide, maybe this disease will kill me instead.

Then I worried it wouldn't, because I wanted out.

I don't want to be in this state anymore.

Every day I was so *tired*. I had no idea what fatigue was until I got this sick.

Fatigue was waking up and not being able to get out of bed until 12:00 p.m. But before I could set one foot on the floor, from 9:00 a.m. to 12:00 p.m., I literally said to myself, *Get up*. I talked to myself and tried to get up for three hours straight. It *might* work by 12:00 p.m. I might get out of bed. But it didn't work every day.

Every part of me wanted to die. Death made sense. I made plans and looked up elaborate ways to do it. One day when I fell into sleep, I hallucinated.

I can't believe this. I'm literally seeing and hearing voices.

The voices were entities in my room.

I'm tripping hard.

But I couldn't share my experience with anyone.

They'll think I have gone insane.

But then I realized...

I HAVE gone insane.

I was losing my mind. I was losing my memories. Matt was worried because whenever we talked on the phone, I couldn't remember anything. I didn't get his references or stories about stuff we'd done together.

What the fuck. I didn't even know these mental states existed.

One day my brain fog was so severe, I felt mentally disabled.

No, I am mentally disabled.

It's time to end my suffering.

I got on the computer and looked up "how to buy a gun in California," but I couldn't understand the instructions or what I was reading. I could see the words, but they didn't string together or make sense.

Holy shit, I can't understand the written word. I'm so sick I can't even figure out how to buy a gun to kill myself.

It was the ultimate prison. Not only was I locked in a prison, I couldn't even escape it by suicide.

I reached out to my friend Jeremy. This was hard to do. I didn't want to admit I was sick. I didn't want to admit I was weak—and I looked at asking for help as being weak. But I had hit a breaking point where I didn't care what somebody thought. I didn't care if people knew I wasn't doing well.

Jeremy told me about a good therapist he used to see, so I booked a session.

Dr. Allman's office was in an old-fashioned area of El Cajon. His room had a mix of outdated and newer books and toys. The vibe was old-school, although this therapist was up to date on the techniques of the day. He had white hair and an attitude that he had seen a lot of stuff, but he still loved you either way. It was an "I love you but don't feed me any bullshit" attitude, which was perfect. Being there reminded me of the theme of *Good Will Hunting*. Matt Damon's character is super messed up. His therapist has to drop traditional techniques to try to get through to him. I was a super messed up person, and there was this therapist who, for whatever reason, wanted to help me—just like in the movie.

I explained that I had Lyme, that I wanted to die, and that I thought about suicide all the time. As I spoke, I knew it was risky to admit that. By law, therapists have to report if you are at risk of harming yourself or others. Still, I shared it all. The therapist knew what was up and that I had to share it with him but that I wasn't going to end my life. He made sure I was OK to share what was truly going on, and I didn't have to worry about him reporting me for sharing my true thoughts.

"I need two sessions per week."

"You want to meet two times per week?" Dr. Allman furrowed his brow with curiosity and concern.

"Yes."

"Any particular reason?"

"If I don't, I will kill myself."

He stared straight at me as if he wanted to make sure I was as serious as I was. Ten seconds went by.

"Let's do Mondays and Thursdays. Does that work?"

We did intense EMDR sessions.

EMDR stands for "eye movement desensitization and reprocessing." It's a psychotherapy treatment used to treat unprocessed trauma and PTSD. It's not entirely accepted in psychotherapy circles, and it's not entirely clear how it works. The therapy itself involves bilateral stimulation (like moving the eyes back and forth) while thinking about traumatic events. The way we did it, I got alternating sounds in my ears, while also feeling pulses in devices I held in my hands. I had plenty of traumatic events to think about, past and present. Supposedly, EMDR helps process that trauma and rewire the brain to be healthier. I had a lot of issues around loss and abandonment in addition to the enormous physical and mental toll my illnesses were taking on me.

This felt like hard-core therapy. I was able to tell him everything I was going through, which I'd really hesitated to do with friends (because I was afraid I'd scare them away) and couldn't do with business colleagues (because I felt I couldn't show weakness) or with family members (because they couldn't be there for me).

After my brother Nathan died in 2006, my family fell apart. I didn't talk to my dad, Jim, much. I hardly talked to my mom, Christena. My older sister, Natalie, seemed distant—she didn't talk to any of us. My younger brother, Brady, was super young and was not equipped to deal with something that traumatic.

If one of us called another, the conversation would be about surface-level topics. We'd talk about a basketball game or something. Our relationships weren't bad, but they weren't deep. They weren't really supportive relationships. For a while I tried to bring everyone together, even tried to get everyone into therapy, but eventually, I gave up.

It would have been nice to have an actual family where we had each others' backs. Instead, we all were trying to survive on our own; that was our way of handling Nathan's death. I get that we were all hurt people just doing our best.

Dr. Allman and I created family figures within my brain. I constructed the perfect parental figure, who I could access to hug me when I needed it. I cried and mourned the loss of my life. I mourned the loss of my childhood best friend, Spencer, who had died suddenly from a seizure; I looked deep into my family and connection issues; I did everything I could to work out all my bullshit.

I had worked so hard to compartmentalize my life so I could function. Those EMDR sessions were the only place where I could feel certain emotions like sadness and despair and loneliness. I don't think anyone in my family had set out to ignore me or abandon me during this time of Lyme suffering—they just didn't know what was truly going on with me and didn't go out of their way to find out.

I still wanted to kill myself. I saw this therapist for eight months straight. The bizarre but intense EMDR I was doing twice a week was the only thing keeping me alive. I still had suicidal ideations, but they didn't get worse. I could deal with them.

* * *

During this time, I was still doing improv and even making some friends in class. My friend Alan and I did a couple of open mics in between our stand-up comedy classes, even though I was scared shitless.

When we scheduled our first stand-up show at the Comedy Palace club, I couldn't think straight. Although I was onstage five times per week through improv and my stand-up comedy class, anxiety plagued me for days before the show.

Sometimes, when I got up onstage in class, I would be so nervous that I couldn't remember anything at all. I knew that I had to completely memorize everything from my tonality to my body movements to my delivery; it all had to be planned perfectly and cemented into my unconscious memory. If not, I would be too fucked to perform.

I practiced relentlessly, doing my set so many times I lost count. My days were consumed with practicing because my anxiety had me so wound up and convinced that I would mess it up once I got up there.

The night before my show, I took a bunch of sleep meds and supplements to try to sleep, but Lyme already had me in the grips of anxiety. Combine that with stage fright and the fear of performing my first show, and I didn't sleep well. Then I was worried my sleep deprivation would mess me up even more onstage.

When I woke up, I was nervous as all hell. I brewed some Sleepy-time tea, then got anxious it would make me too drowsy and mess up my performance. I took some caffeine, but that made me afraid the caffeine would give me more anxiety. This led to some chamomile tea and having to piss every ten minutes from all the liquid I was pregaming with.

When I finally got onstage at the Comedy Palace, I was so nervous that my hand holding the mic was shaking, but I knew nobody could tell. In my sales experience, I learned that people can't tell what's going on inside; they can only see the exterior. Your exterior gives away far less than you think it does. Although now my exterior was shaking and giving my secret anxiety away, I told people I was too far away for them to see that. That made me feel a little better.

Trying to stay alive made me develop a darker sense of humor. My routine that night included a Lyme bit at the end. I had to make fun of what I was feeling. If I didn't, I couldn't cope. I put it in there because it's hard to accept a serious medical diagnosis of yourself. Other people might not hold a stigma against you, but you will hold it against yourself—and that pushes people away.

I was having a hard time accepting that I had Lyme disease, so I used stand-up comedy to cope with it. When I turned a segment of my performance into jokes about Lyme, it entertained the audience, but I really included it to heal myself.

"I got to move to San Diego where all the best doctors are," I said from the stage. "Plus, in Texas, they kept asking me how many guys I had unprotected sex with—it has nothing to do with Lyme!

"Two, all it means is I feel horrible and shallow on the inside, but I still look good on the outside. So when I moved to Southern California I just fit right in!"

That line got me a lot of laughs.

"But the best part is dating was instantly enhanced because it lowers your libido, so I last forever. So on my dating profile I put, 'Once you go Lyme, you're gonna get plenty of time.'"

People laughed at that one too.

"I'm getting all these messages and they're coming over, but they didn't know what Lyme was. They thought it was actually *limes*, so they're bringing all these limes. The other thing is Lyme makes these weird marks on your skin; they thought that was because I was getting whipped or something.

"So there are limes everywhere, they're rubbing lime on me and putting salt on it, licking it off, and getting all kinky. I'm going whoa, this is a new world for Taylor James, mmm, tastes so good!"

During this last bit, I rubbed an actual lime on my body, then threw it out to the crowd. It hit someone in the chest and splashed their drink.

Although I hate watching myself, the performance is here if you want to check it out:

I felt alive after my set. It was healing to see people laugh and accept the Lyme part of me. What's funny is that people *will* accept you for all the parts you accept of yourself. But people won't accept what you don't accept. I was having a hard time accepting Lyme.

After that first show, someone offered me the chance to perform at the Mad House Comedy Club, which felt badass. Fresh off my performance, I was able to get right back up onstage again. I credit the Cumanda I had taken. For some reason, that herb sometimes made me feel functional for a day or two.

My second show felt flawless. It was the most surreal feeling. I had never been onstage with absolute confidence and zero fear. A combination of just coming off that first show and having the right tincture gave me the relief I needed. Onstage, I kept eye contact with the audience and had complete control over them. As my parting gift to them, once again, I rubbed a lime on my body and threw it into the crowd.

I had told people from that stage that I looked normal on the outside, even though I felt horrible on the inside. But after those shows, I actually felt good on the inside—for a little while.

That weekend I went to a party hosted by a mastermind group. I was so alive and felt so good off the show that I started hitting everyone up, using my stand-up comedy jokes and routine. Everyone loved it. I felt I made friends with every woman there.

But I'd overplayed my hand. The mastermind group leader called to say I wasn't going to be accepted in the group because I "hit on too many women." I hadn't realized what I was doing at the time.

I'd just been so happy that I was talking to everyone, but someone didn't like that. I was banned from that mastermind group.

Then a friend who was in that group told me he couldn't be around me anymore because I had Lyme. According to him, I must've had bad vibrational thoughts to attract something like that. He strongly believed in the book *The Secret* and told me that I had to change my thoughts to get better. He was actually saying that I'd attracted Lyme, that it was my fault I'd gotten it. He said since my vibrations were off, being around me was bad for him. People who told me stuff like this made me crazy—they had no idea what I was dealing with.

Then another friend, who had invited me to the mastermind group in the first place, told me something similar. He said it wasn't healthy for him to be around me. I had taught him everything he knew about sales, but he didn't feel any obligation to stick with me. What I was going through was too heavy, he said, and I wasn't emotionally healthy.

I'd felt so confident after those two comedy shows. I felt I had made a small comeback, but I guess my brain was still broken. I wasn't all there after all. Just when I'd thought I might actually gain a tribe or a social circle to be a part of—something I so desperately wanted—I was shunned. I know now that these were transactional friends, not real friends. But the rejection hurt.

I was on an emotional and physical roller coaster, from the high of performance—which I loved—to experiencing even more despair. The people who I had gone to the ends of the earth for were abandoning me.

I didn't know how to move forward with stand-up, so I just quit. I stopped working on it entirely.

Stand-up and improv performances provided me with momentary escapes from suffering. When I had a good day, the relief was amazing. Simply feeling normal felt like living life on easy mode. Being back to your true self for one day is like being on cocaine, ecstasy, and mushrooms all at once. That's how happy you get when you feel any sort of reprieve from the physical agony, although I've never done that combination of drugs so if you have, please tell me if that's accurate.

I took advantage of any fleeting moment of relief. Once, when I suddenly had a bit of energy, I ran from the hallway and dove onto my bed, then I would run back again, leaping further and further each time to see how far I could land. My roommate couldn't stop laughing as I couldn't get enough of running back and forth just to jump onto my bed.

But the lows were worsening. My life was still deteriorating every day. Some days were worse than others, but they were all pretty shitty.

My joints started to hurt, which was never my main Lyme symptom. My neck was so stiff I couldn't turn it. Anyone with Lyme reading this who has had the "stiff neck" knows what I am talking about. The pain behind my eyes was a weird constant pressure, like a headache but not. My brain fog felt like I was trying to drive from LA to New York with three feet of visibility in front of me. I was so tired that brushing my teeth felt like running ten miles. My anxiety was so bad that I couldn't make friends. I was handicapped and limited.

There was a beautiful beach ten minutes away from my place, and I almost never went. That's right. I can count on one hand the number of times I went to the beach while I lived in San Diego.

* * *

Bartonella can cause rage.[1] Of all the tick-borne diseases, it's the one that really did a number on me. That, plus all the crap I was experiencing, produced some interesting moments.

I was walking in the Gaslamp Quarter one day when I went off on someone who looked at me weird. I almost fought him. This was a random stranger on the street. But I had nothing to lose. I was so angry that I couldn't think clearly. And I had no fear because I didn't care if I died. The other guy wouldn't fight. He must've seen that I had lost my mind, and he didn't want to engage.

Afterward, I realized that rage felt better than being complacent and depressed, but it could lead to serious consequences. Still thinking about the almost-fight, I went off on a weird little tangent and researched the legalities of fighting. I learned that it's illegal even if both parties agree to it. My searches led me to a book called *The Little Black Book of Violence.* I read most of it to try to convince myself not to have these types of confrontations anymore. It worked. The book taught me that no matter what, when you fight, nobody wins. Even if you do technically win, if you keep doing it, you will eventually get permanently hurt or

---

1 Lyme has been documented to cause rage, "homicidality," and a lot of other awful tendencies, according to a study conducted by the National Institutes of Health. Robert C. Bransfield, "Aggressiveness, violence, homicidality, homicide, and Lyme disease," *Neuropsychiatric Disease and Treatment* 14 (March 9, 2018): 693–713, https://www.ncbi.nlm.nih.gov/pmc/articles/PMC5851570/.

have serious legal issues. If I went to prison, I'd be screwed. Last time I checked, there aren't any healthy foods, infrared saunas, or supplements in there.

I was doing everything I could to make sure my rageful self wouldn't do that again. I had read that Lyme could cause rage, abrupt mood swings, poor impulse control, psychosis, paranoia, explosive anger, and more. That didn't make actually dealing with all of that any easier. My fucked-up mind couldn't help but think fighting would be a fun way to die. Fighting someone in the street and dying would be better than hanging or shooting myself. The thoughts of suicide got louder and louder. I needed to die. There was no point in being alive.

One of the big problems with Lyme-induced mental illness is you don't know that the Lyme is causing it. Your doctor or therapist might not know either, especially if you haven't been diagnosed with Lyme. Bartonella can literally change who you are, which is absolutely creepy.

Most people don't understand suicide. They think the person who took their life was selfish for leaving everyone else behind. They think the person was weak and a wuss for taking the "easy way" out. They think the person was an idiot.

If God had come into my room and told me that no matter what, I would never feel better than how I was feeling at that point for the rest of my life, I would have ended my life. There would be no point to live like that with no hope of ever getting better.

Trust me. Nobody who's stared into Satan's eyes while in the depths of hell for months on end in pure suffering thinks they are taking the easy way out. I saw a therapist twice a week for the *sole* purpose of *not* killing myself, and I was *still* about to do it.

At one point I thought, *My entire life could be suffering, but I have to carry on.* I went back and forth like this in my head until I was so overwhelmed that my brain tipped toward the suicide solution; one day in early February 2017 I texted Cody: "I can't take it anymore, and I'm going to kill myself." Then I went to sleep.

When I woke up in the morning, I saw that Cody had called over and over. When he called again, I answered, thinking he was probably worried that I was going to commit suicide.

"Hey, TJ." His voice was devoid of emotion.

"Man, I'm sorry about that text last night. You're probably worried about that."

"Carlos finally did himself in. He took his life last night."

"Wait, what?"

"Yeah. I guess he took a bunch of pills and drank alcohol and never woke up."

"Fuck. I guess this means I'm flying to Utah."

"I'll see you there."

Goddammit.

There I was, about to kill myself, when one of my best friends, Carlos, took his own life. Carlos and I had met in high school. He was funny and nonjudgmental and loving. No matter what was going on, he'd start joking around and make me feel better. After my brother Nathan died he helped me a lot. I even lived at his house for a while. He was one of the best people in my life.

And now he was gone.

In the past, he had sat in his garage with the car on and had taken a bunch of pills. He'd also threatened to off himself multiple times. *This time he went through with it.* His wife had cheated on him and asked for a divorce, which had devastated him. He'd felt like his family was ruined. It's hard to say if he'd been committed to actually killing himself that night or if he had been simply depressed and only trying to hurt himself. Either way, he was gone.

Carlos's death took a lot out of me. My body broke down harder from stress. Emotions, for me, translated into physical stress, which could leave me feeling wrecked. To prevent that I had to prevent myself from feeling a lot of normal emotions. I lived in a suppressed state, just trying to hold it together. The emotional burden of Carlos's death was another weight on top of what I was carrying, and it broke me physically.

Everyone who knew Carlos in Utah was devastated, but I was strong for them. I stayed positive when I was around others. I offered support. I hung out and made jokes. I tried to help out. I'm not sure why, but that's just what I do. I try to have big enough shoulders for everyone. Paradoxically, even though I felt horrible and had contemplated taking my life right before his death, I was the rock. Carlos had just beaten me to it.

To remember him, some of Carlos's family and friends and I got his fingerprint on a dog tag. I wear it every day.

I was shattered inside, but everyone back in Utah only saw my strong external shell. I believed I had to earn love, and being able to support others was one way I could do that. When they depended on me it made me feel they wouldn't leave me. Since I get importance from being people's rock, I liked that feeling.

No one at the funeral could tell how sick I was, just like the audience at my show couldn't tell how nervous I was, and just like my clients in Texas couldn't tell how stressed out or intimidated I was when pitching them solar.

Remember, people can only see the outside. They can't see the inside.

Someone once said that "everyone is fighting their own battle." You never *really* know the struggles others are facing. You are only getting a glimpse. When you are interacting with someone, you are dipping your toe two inches into a fifteen-foot-deep pool of who they *really* are and what they are *really* going through.

CHAPTER
6

"Of all the things I've lost, I miss my mind the most."

—MARK TWAIN

WHEN I RETURNED TO SAN DIEGO, I COLLAPSED. MORE and more marks appeared on my skin from coinfections. I joined two acting classes but dropped out of one because I wasn't feeling it. I wanted to be savage, and it was too contained for me. I lived such a compartmentalized life, I kept my emotions so suppressed, that I knew I needed some sort of outlet, and I wanted acting to be it.

So I went to another super intense acting class in a different part of town. That one focused on what we were feeling. It was so emotional trying to be...emotional. I was not comfortable with my emotions, but acting was where I was supposed to explore emotions. Precisely because it was hard, I was attracted to it. I lived with so much daily emotional chaos that I knew I needed to get a handle on it. I needed an outlet. This was the perfect challenge.

Maybe I'll be an actor!

I had brain fog to the extent that I was mentally handicapped, and I was confused as hell. I didn't know what to do. I didn't know where to direct my energies in any area of my life. Whatever popped into my brain seemed like a viable choice. I would leap into action spurred by random thoughts and urges. I did whatever I could to escape the pain.

One day, in my acting class, we did an exercise.

"If you are feeling real emotion, then you are not 'acting,'" the instructor said. In other words, if you are giving a true performance, you will actually experience it within you. The goal of acting was to make it feel real to yourself, so it was no longer "acting." It would then be real for the audience.

He told us to bring something that was very important to us to the next class. The thing I needed to bring was already with me— Carlos's dog tag. When it was hard to do something, and it took all my willpower, I would hold my necklace and tell myself, *Do it for Carlos*. This necklace was my lifeline.

The acting exercise went like this: Two people worked together. One handed over the valuable item, and then had to convince the other to return it. Only when the other person felt real emotions coming from the other actor could they return the object. If they felt you weren't fully experiencing your feelings in the moment, they were to hold onto your important item.

My anxiety shot through the roof as I watched others try and fail to retrieve their valuables. While I waited my turn, I thought, *I use this necklace to get up in the morning. Without it, I might not have gone on. If my friend hadn't died, I might have taken my own life.*

Nobody was getting their item back. Then it was my turn. I handed my necklace to my partner, a Goth, bubbly woman who held it behind her back.

"May I have my necklace back?" I asked.

"No."

"I REALLY need that back," I said, a little more intensely.

"I don't believe you."

I asked for it back over and over, my voice growing louder and louder.

The acting coach told me that more volume didn't make my emotions more real. I went soft and earnest. Whispering didn't do the trick either.

My face was flushed and hot, my hands sweating. My life flashed before my eyes. *I need my dead friend's necklace. I need that shit back. Give me my fucking friend's necklace back.*

"You are never going to get this back."

I responded suddenly without thinking about it, "You DON'T UNDERSTAND...I NEED THAT NECKLACE." I started crying while I stared into her eyes. I knew from the way her expression changed that she felt all the pain in my life boil over. Everything spilled out. My external shell shattered, so there was no longer a barrier between my inner and outer worlds. Both worlds aligned as the entire room got a taste of my pure Lyme suffering. Of my shit existence.

Tears rolled down my face, and my partner cried with me. She handed me my necklace and said, "Wow...you were the only one to pass the test." The acting coach sat in silence as he observed what had happened, and I took my seat, my walls coming back up as I closed off again.

Yes, I was the only one to pass the test, but from that one encounter, I was wiped out for four days.

That was it. I had wanted to be savage, but I couldn't handle the emotional stress of acting. I emailed the instructor to tell him I couldn't make it to the classes anymore.

* * *

Without acting, I needed something to bring me back to life. I messaged a guy I'd heard about who knew how to use Rife machines. A Rife machine is a device that delivers low-energy electromagnetic frequency into the body. Different frequencies are supposed to help with different ailments.

He invited me over to his home on the second level of an apartment building in Ocean Beach. When I arrived, he was talking to a woman, about the age of thirty-five, who I thought must have Lyme too. Her skin was unhealthy. Some people with Lyme have a certain tight and dry texture to their skin as if they are dehydrated, only they aren't. I've only seen women affected by it.

I knew from her face that this woman was suffering, but she still smiled like she had hope as she held a jarful of kefir, which is a fermented dairy product, sort of like thick milk. I figured the Rife guy helped people by giving them kefir grains in addition to treating them with the machine.

He showed me a Spooky Rife—a certain model of the machine. We dialed in the frequencies for what would be most effective for me after he asked me a series of questions about which pathogens I had and what symptoms I was struggling with.

While I was using the Rife machine and the bulb was flickering on and off, I couldn't tell if I felt anything. Still, we sat there as he entertained me with the story of the person who invented it and how subsequent promoters had been prosecuted for fraud, yet he believed that the Rife machine could cure cancer, and so on. He also showed me how he'd built a Rife machine. He explained to me about the orb, a cylinder in a circle with all sorts of wires surrounding it. It looked angelical because it was so symmetrical, like something inspired by a higher power.

I could see he had gone off the deep end and had become totally obsessed with beating Lyme with Rife machines. The question I couldn't ignore in my head was, *If Rife machines work so well, why is this man still sick with Lyme?*

I could tell he simply loved to try to help people, and he wasn't motivated at all by money. What he did came from his heart.

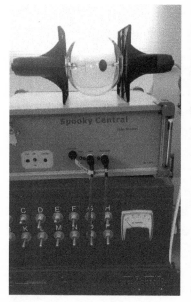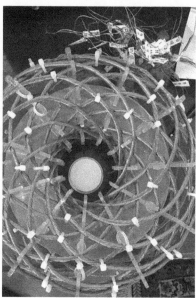

"I work off donations," he told me. I wasn't ready to buy into the Rife hype, but I did give him twenty bucks.

* * *

It makes sense to me now that some of the best creatives are the most internally tortured. Sure, some good stuff comes out of blissful and happy states, but true art representing the human condition arises out of deep suffering. My life had come down to trying to distract myself before joining Carlos in the afterlife.

I needed an outlet to cope. During one of my mini mental breakdowns late at night, I wrote a Lyme rap.

I'll start singing songs and rapping music to crowds. That's how I'll make it.

I had plans for performing live, another way to escape my suffering by being onstage. I put a beat to it, planning it out in my head to become a whole music video. My wireless speaker was ready to go. I memorized all the lines and searched for open mic nights so I could perform it.

Lyme Mind

They say no pain, no gain

But I'm sitting here daily feeling like my mind's going insane

It's weird how the news doesn't let it get any fame

It's scary how many people out there with the Lyme brain

You think of big things like maybe I'll be an actor

One audition leaves you like you've been run over by a tractor

You thought you could make it despite Borrelia's negative factors

Your only escape is dark humor, dark laughter

You reach for your goals, but your body says no

Killing coinfections with the oil of oregano

The next day your energy has come to a close

You won't even be able to change a simple laundry load

People make plans that you have to avoid

Who knows if you'll wake up that morning and feel destroyed

People with disease, my heart goes out to you

That brain fog makes it hard to figure out what to do

People playing basketball working on their shootin'

But you're just worried that you're gonna die from eating gluten

Living with an invisible, secretive, internal hell

But at least you still look good on your outward, external shell

You hope it can be curable, but only time will tell

You wonder how you ever took for granted feeling well

Sometimes you're put on your crackling knees

Begging for mercy and thinking, please

Any good day is a glimpse and a tease

When your body has made friends with this Lyme disease

Had to stop lifting and let your body go weak

Don't even plan on a night of good sleep

Knowing when you take your shirt off at the nearby park

People see cat-scratch fever's made its mark

Almost two years with symptoms asking what is it?

All these doctors want over five hundred bucks per visit

You spend your life researching almost every single minute

You wish you could just get cured at one magical clinic

Healing takes years and years of perfect technique

In the middle of the journey and the mind can go weak

When you're looking for sanity but it's playing hide-and-seek

Your kitchen has transformed into a supplement boutique

Think and Grow Rich *and* The Secret *all the time*

But all that fake positive thinking doesn't make you feel fine

Blaming yourself for attracting a tick is a mental crime

It just stresses you out and makes you Think and Grow Lyme

Pain still exists on medical marijuana

Looking up prices for ozone in Tijuana

Shit isn't cheap reaching a zone of health nirvana

No couch in my living room, just an infrared sauna

CHAPTER
7

"One of the hardest decisions you'll ever face in life is choosing whether to walk away or try harder."

—ZIAD K. ABDELNOUR

ONE NIGHT MY FRIEND JEFF INVITED ME TO MEET WITH him and some people in Little Italy, a place in San Diego known for its lack of parking. Whenever I'm in that area, I have a rule— if I am within three blocks of my destination and I see a parking spot, I take it. I don't wait to see if I can find something better. As I drove the same streets repeatedly, my senses turned on high alert.

I looked for parking for about ten minutes. Most people would have kept hunting, especially if others were waiting for you and you'd already driven twenty minutes to the location. But this time, I didn't care. I told Jeff that I'd catch up with him tomorrow. Then I turned around, drove home, and laid down instead. I couldn't handle the stress of *finding a parking space.*

My stress tolerance lessened; my ability to converse lessened. I was just a shell of who I used to be. I'm not religious, and I'm not sure why I felt compelled to pray, but the pain all over my body and the pain from the sheer exhaustion of living got so intense that some nights I dropped to my knees and prayed. I leaned my elbows on the bed and sat there in the prayer position for twenty minutes or more. The agony was so unbearable that I, a nonreligious person, would fall to my knees and pray.

I still had friends, though, and I am forever appreciative of them.

I met Alan and Justin M. at improv classes, and we hung out and built memories together. My friend Jeff, who I have known for a long time, is a high-level human being in every sense of the word and didn't seem to care that I bailed due to the parking situation. I would invite him over to partake in a "kratom shrine" where I would make a cup of kratom on the counter surrounded by two crystals, just because it was funny to exaggerate the whole spiritual healing scenario. (Kratom is a plant derivative that seems to affect the opioid receptors in the brain and works like a pain killer.)

My friend Cody was just a phone call away. Trey in Utah was a lifelong friend who wasn't going anywhere. Jonny was a friend who was there during both the highs and the lows.

It takes special friends to look at the person behind the illness, to still see that human. If I were on the other side, a healthy person looking in at my sick self, it wouldn't be easy to decipher what was going on. I wondered what some people saw when they looked at me.

People are usually confused when they look at me, because I feel I am in a prison, but the bars are invisible. As I said during my stand-up routine, I look good on the outside. It confuses people when you explain how much you are hurting but look great. The only time I could show people externally what was happening on the inside was when I was getting rashes—still, you don't necessarily want to whip those out.

Of course, there are people who don't believe what you are saying. These people don't understand. They think your prison bars are an illusion that the mind can overcome with willpower, that health issues can be fixed overnight with the proper mindset and positive thinking.

"But you look so good," they'd tell me. "You look healthy. I'm sure you can get over it."

One friend told me to listen to some hypnosis tapes while I went to sleep at night, and in three to five days, I would be cured of Lyme. That sort of goofball suggestion was common—especially years ago when Lyme was less well-publicized. It was really frustrating to be treated that way.

None of that works.

It's a bit bizarre that this belief in the overriding power of the mind exists, but I believe that is because there *are* certain things that can be flipped around with willpower. Procrastination, mild depression, garden-variety sadness, thought loops, etc., all can be overcome to a degree. After all, I began my fight with Lyme convinced that I could win through willpower and character. But an illness is way more complex than that. Lyme affects the brain, the tool itself that these people told me I should use to overcome my illness.

You would never tell someone who cut their finger off that they didn't need to go to the hospital—that they could simply use their thoughts to heal their finger. In the same way, you can't will your way to stopping a spirochete from invading every crevice of your body. The main thing that a proper mindset can do is help keep your stress levels down, so your body can be in a healing state.

No matter how much I tried to explain this, people who were big into the "power of the mind" still left me.

I'm not saying that mindset isn't important. It is. But maybe it is about 30 percent of the equation when healing a serious illness like Lyme. I am not discounting that my mindset helped me to a degree, but most of what helped was physical treatments.

I got used to compartmentalizing everything, from the pain to the suffering to the fatigue. I started to break myself into different parts so I could function. I had to turn off, otherwise I would never survive all the trauma. Living with Lyme is like being traumatized every single day for years on end. For instance, I might wake up and see a red mark on my stomach from Bartonella. A normal person would freak out, figure out what was going on, reschedule their day to take care of themselves. I couldn't afford to do any of that. I'd just note the mark and try to keep going with my day. I'd tell myself, "I won't think about that." I couldn't allow myself to feel the full extent of it, or it would be over.

I suppressed everything. Just chopped it up into pieces and stuffed it away. Being sick taught me to turn it off. The way my body turned negative emotions into physical pain *forced* me to turn it off. The only time I dealt with my emotions was during my fifty-minute EMDR sessions with the therapist I was still seeing twice a week.

* * *

In addition to the mental war games that Lyme plays, you have to be almost perfect every single day when you have this disease. If you don't go to bed on time, if you eat the wrong thing, if you don't take your supplements, if you don't meditate, if you don't watch your thoughts, if you don't handle your stress and emotions properly, if you don't keep tabs on when to reorder supplements and medications, if you don't connect with people to avoid depression, if you don't get the proper testing and track your symptoms, if you just barely slip up at all...it's game over.

After striving for this level of perfection day in and day out, every now and then, I would lose my mind. I'd be perfect for five weeks in a row, then suddenly, I'd say, "Fuck it!" I'd get kombucha alcohol, some sugar cake thing from Sprouts, and put porn on without even really watching it because I was completely losing my libido.

Or I would take a bunch of drugs and wander around my neighborhood. I just needed some kind of relief.

One night, I lost my mind. I took a bunch of marijuana, ripped off my shirt, grabbed a Bluetooth speaker, and longboarded at high speeds around my neighborhood while dancing on the board. I went back and forth, staying close to my house so I didn't get lost (I didn't trust my brain to find the way home).

I kept passing one house that had the blinds up. They must've been watching me as I kept cruising by, blasting my music and dancing around, all by myself.

It hit me then that I was THAT crazy person. I was the deranged dude that you see outside on a random street, the one who you stay away from. You know that you will not be able to connect with them because they are in some alternate reality. You know they are lonely too. You don't want to engage. If you do, they will talk your ear off with no social awareness that you don't care...I was that person now.

People thought I was gone...but even knowing that I still didn't give a shit. When people say they don't care what other people think, there's a 99 percent chance they still do. It's the 1 percent of motherfuckers who have hit a point of no return and cannot give a shit who truly don't. That's not a pretty place to be. It's good to give a shit a little bit.

* * *

After this new batch of mini mental breakdowns subsided, I started to question if the Cowden Protocol—a series of herbs like Banderol, Cumanda, Pinella, Houttuynia, etc.—was actually working to kill my Lyme and coinfections. I started following it when I started working with Dr. Casey from Idaho. He tried to time my taking them at certain intervals when rashes or symptoms appeared in specific ways. Testing showed elevated levels of ALT (alanine transaminase, an enzyme) in my liver, which could have meant liver damage; high monocytes that indicated an active infection; high eosinophils, which showed I had inflammation; and low testosterone at 380, about half what I should have.

Despite taking and doing everything this doctor was telling me to, I was getting worse every day. One day, in an effort to feel better, I said *screw it* and sprayed a bunch of marijuana oil under my tongue; I took a large spoonful of kratom and randomly went to a library. It was full of people who weren't all there mentally and had clearly seen rough times. I thought to myself, *I fit in here.*

I used to feel a bit uncomfortable in a library full of homeless people and "broken" characters. Not because I don't like those kinds of people or would judge them, but because I don't want to engage in rambling, inescapable conversations that start if I make eye contact. This time, I was comfortable; this time, people didn't want to engage with *me*.

I picked up a book by Richard I. Horowitz called *Why Can't I Get Better?* The marijuana spray kicked in, and the kratom numbed my pain. Surprisingly, this drug combination allowed me to understand the book, and I sat still long enough to digest the information. As I lost myself in the book, I realized that it had been a long time since I had experienced the dopamine rush that happens when reading and neural connections form as new thoughts and knowledge take root. Now, that feeling was suddenly accessible again because I was high.

The book discussed antibiotics and how a lot of Lyme patients can't get better with one approach. Horowitz argued that some people could improve with herbal treatments, and some couldn't. Maybe my opposition to antibiotics was wrong. My overall Lyme situation was not improving. Maybe the natural route wasn't going to work. I read at the library for six hours and left with new ideas for the future brewing in my brain.

I called Dr. Casey in Idaho and went over a few things. Based on my symptoms and current rash (my rashes cycled in and out in different forms back then), he reluctantly agreed that I should go on a two-week cycle of doxycycline. I asked him if it was normal to take this antibiotic at this late stage of the Lyme game, as I had only heard of it being prescribed for freshly bitten people. Antibiotics can kill Lyme right away if you take them as soon as you are bitten, so it never develops into a long-term problem. How could doxycycline possibly work in just two weeks at this stage? He assured me that doxy is so strong a two-week hit would be enough. I got the prescription.

When I first took doxycycline the effect was intense. I started getting a terrible Herxheimer reaction. This is what happens when you kill off a lot of Lyme pathogens. Your body can become very inflamed as it tries to detoxify all the dead Lyme spirochetes. I felt like there were knife blades in my stomach, and I was shitting them out in my diarrhea three to four times per day. I tried to take extra detox baths, but they just weren't doing it.

After nearly a week of this, I started to feel better. My mind cleared up some and I had more energy.

Oh nice, I'm starting to get some relief!

I could get a few things done around the house. Then my two-week cycle ran out. When I stopped the antibiotic, everything stopped.

The relief stopped.

The energy stopped.

Deep depression sank its hooks into me. I felt more horrible than before I started the doxy. Once again, I felt I couldn't take it anymore. I told my therapist that I couldn't make it in that week. And I was done working with Dr. Casey.

I don't give a shit.

Fuck all this.

This is it.

I'm done.

Once again, I researched all the ways to end my life (other than buying a gun, because that's too hard and complicated in California). When I woke up one morning, I knew how to do it. I concluded that jumping from a bridge would be the easiest way to go. Here's the logical way a suicidal person's mind works:

- I wouldn't have to explain to a store why I needed multiple containers of helium gas, so I could fill up my room, pass out, and asphyxiate.

- I didn't have to get a gun and worry that I wouldn't do it right, let alone figure out how to obtain the firearm in the first place. Not to mention it would be horrific for whoever would find me. I didn't want someone to go through that.

- Hanging seemed too grotesque, and I didn't want to resist it once it started—as well as I didn't want to be found like that either.

- Other methods seemed a bit too violent and painful.

- But jumping off a bridge...all I had to do was take one step forward and plunge to my death.

I had watched the movie *The Bridge* multiple times. It was about people who committed suicide by jumping off of the Golden Gate Bridge. I knew the only thing that would suck about the bridge option was changing my mind after I jumped. Survivors always say that as soon as their decision is irreversible, they wish they hadn't jumped. But the irreversible part is what would be the trick.

I looked up the Coronado Bridge, took a screenshot of it, and sent it to a couple of people, letting them know I'd had enough. This was finally it.

Then...instead of driving over to the bridge, I forgot I even sent the texts and what my plans were. I guess my brain fog blotted it out. I ignored my phone and carried on with the next task of my life. I got in a detox bath, where I lay for hours.

Until I met Officer Joseph Smith and his partners from the San Diego Police Department.

* * *

After I talked my way out of the psychiatric hospital, my friend Matt showed up—just like he'd promised that doctor he would.

We hung out for a couple days, but I knew I had to make a change. It was time to go home to Utah to try to heal. My friend Justin R. and his wife, Ashlee, who had a place in River-dale, Utah, told me I could crash in their basement until I got settled. I was and am forever grateful for that. We don't talk much anymore, but their gesture still holds a special place in my heart.

I tried to return the infrared sauna to Jeff. He told me to pay what I owed on the rent—$600—and keep it. Jeff had beaten cancer when he was younger. Whenever someone has had a really bad illness, they understand when another person is fighting for their life. That infrared sauna was thousands of dollars new, and I could have sold it for more than that used. Jeff hooked it up for me. He wanted to pay it forward.

I rented a U-Haul truck and hooked my car up behind it. I looked at the trailer for the car and knew that it would be a pain in the ass to manage, then went to bed. After about three hours of sleep, I woke up because my Lyme was inflamed. My feet burned, my body ached, and there was pain behind my eyes. I was utterly exhausted.

Holy shit, I have to drive this thing back to Utah.

It was hard enough driving in general with Lyme in California traffic. Now, I had to drive a massive U-Haul while sleep-de-prived, sick as hell from Lyme, and with twelve hours of drive time ahead of me. And I had to get gas! Filling that monstrous rig up in a crowded gas station was the most stressful refueling experience I've ever had.

I gripped the steering wheel tightly and I used all my willpower to focus. I had to keep my eyes open, keep my mind free from distraction, and stop swaying the trailer back and forth.

Only about ten hours left.

The countdown to my new life in Utah had begun.

CHAPTER
8

"I don't fear death. I fear the prologues. The senility and pain. After a few years of that, I assume death presents itself as a holiday at the beach."

—DEAD MAN WALKING

I STARED UP AT THE DIMLY LIT CEILING. LIGHT STILL seeped into my room. The crisp cool air told my body to go to sleep as I lay on the blow-up mattress in the computer room in Justin's basement.

Proper sleep is one of the most important keys for recovery from an illness, and Lyme makes it nearly impossible to sleep right. I always slept with an eye mask and earplugs, so random noises or lights coming in from cars on the street wouldn't wake me up. This night, I didn't put the eye mask on. I didn't put the earplugs in. I just stared at the ceiling.

My body shook and twitched from the pain and trauma. Some nights, as I stared at the ceiling my body would jerk, and I'd rock my head back and forth for up to thirty minutes. I wasn't rocking from my physical symptoms or the neurological problem from the Lyme itself. My body was twitching from the Lyme trauma.

Since I'd had to go into compartmentalization mode for the drive from San Diego, I was still numb. Finally, the thoughts clustered in.

How did I get here?

Am I really in Utah right now?

I'm in the basement of someone's house, at rock bottom, in a place I thought I'd never be again. What the hell is going on?

It was so hard to take in what I was going through, so hard to comprehend the real loss of my mind and my very self, that I would shudder and shake from the pain. I didn't cry, I didn't shout out, I didn't say anything, I didn't reach out to anyone. I suffered alone.

In those moments, I felt I had split into two people, becoming Taylor and TJ, two entities trying to process how my life had become a complete nightmare.

I knew I had to talk to myself. I told myself, "Alright man, I love you. I'll be there if no one else is. I'll be there for you. We gotta do this together. You gotta get up, dude. Let's get up."

I was coaching myself, creating a friend out of myself because I needed the help of a friend so badly. I made a version of myself for myself.

I took my usual backup tinctures: the mixture of herbs, including valerian root, to induce sleep. I call them "backup" because they messed me up pretty bad. But I always had just-in-case medications, tinctures, and strong herbs for nights when I wanted to knock out for at least three hours. In the morning, based on what I took, I knew my body wouldn't rebound well.

* * *

The next morning, I eased myself off the air mattress, climbed the steps out of the basement, and greeted Justin, Ashlee, and their two kids. The kids were amazing. I mimicked doggie sounds for them as we sat there, howling, "arrowwww roowwww." They echoed the sounds back to me. Kids are often a gateway to pure joy and curiosity. You can look at them, with their innocence and fresh minds, and feel like you've gone back in time to when you didn't have severe pain.

I put my tinctures in their cupboard and went grocery shopping. I was basically sensitive to everything. I can't eat gluten, dairy, sugar, corn, rice, or anything processed, and I have to eat low carb; otherwise, the bad gut bacteria will take over my stomach and make me sicker.

I didn't realize it at the time, but my sense of smell had deteriorated. Justin later told me that my tinctures still stank up their cabinet for a month after I left!

It felt good to have the fridge fully loaded with all the food I needed. I hate depending on people and always feel guilty about it, since people have held stuff over my head so they can use it against me later and guilt me into doing them a favor. I don't like accepting help because I don't want to depend on people. The people I depended on growing up abandoned me—they left, or they died. The lesson I learned was not to put myself in a situation where I needed people. There was no way I was going to stay with my friends any longer than I needed to.

I began my search for an apartment and set out in my 2002 Corolla to check out a bunch of places in Salt Lake City.

Utah is a cool place. It just isn't for me, and I never would live there unless I absolutely had to. It's cold and polluted in the winter, and I hate cold. It's too slow-moving for a type A person who wants to get shit done all day every day. When I lived there, I'd call someone up to say, "Hey dude, let's go do this thing," and the response might be, "Oh, that's too far away." It would be fifteen minutes away, but he couldn't be bothered. That was typical, and it made me a little nuts.

I'm also not Mormon, so I don't necessarily fit in with most of the people there. The nice thing about Utah, though, is how laid back it is. People were friendly, and I could strike up conversations with everyone. It was easy to simply walk into apartment buildings and find spots available with negotiation room over how much I would pay in rent. I could tell that Utah was going to be much, much easier for me to handle than the competitive and fast-paced environment of California.

Until I got my own place, I hung out with Justin and Ashlee's family each night. There was something really special about it. The games we played got super intense. One game was called "Would You Rather," and the goal as you played it was to get into the wildest debates. When other people came over, they were shocked at the intensity of our game playing. After the game, we dove into deep philosophical conversations about life. Those were special moments and some of the best times that I remember.

Whenever I saw people and their families having a good time doing something simple like playing a card game, it made me smile on the inside. Relationships were nearly impossible due to my fatigue and Lyme brain, but I still hoped that one day I could create that for myself.

Late in the evenings, I Googled "Lyme success stories" to try to get my mind right. After reading the success story of a guy named Kurt on Reddit, I messaged him and we got on the phone. Anyone else with Lyme is usually willing to talk to you if you reach out to them in a normal way.

Kurt told me about the combinations of antibiotics and medications he was taking from a doctor in Maryland. They got him back to being able to exercise and run his business. He'd never found real success until he was on a specific cocktail that consisted of Coartem, a drug used to treat malaria (he took three rounds of a forty-eight- to seventy-two-hour course); the antibiotic azithromycin; and Biaxin (clarithromycin, another antibiotic) for a year. He had tried the natural tinctures of Banderol, Samento, etc., too, that I was taking, but they never got him anywhere. Now, most days, he forgot that he was even sick.

This further cemented in my brain that antibiotics were the route I most likely had to take to get better. I gathered Kurt's protocols and shared them with my new doctor I found in Utah, Dr. Mortell, who agreed we should give them a try.

CHAPTER
9

"Desperation can make a person do surprising things."

—VERONICA ROTH, ALLEGIANT

THE ONLY COFFEE I DO IS THE KIND I GET TO SHOVE UP my ASS.

I wrote that to make you laugh, but when you get sick enough, and you reach a high enough level of pain, you'll do anything. All my fellow coffee-up-the-ass readers will tell you this fact if you aren't already indulging yourself. I had begun doing near-daily coffee enemas in San Diego. The Gerson Institute in San Diego uses coffee enemas in their treatment for helping people with cancer. It's supposed to help your gallbladder and liver in the detoxification process.

I moved into my new one-bedroom apartment on the fourth floor of 500 West in Salt Lake City. Justin, Ashlee, and my father helped me move in. I wasn't super close with my father, and I was a bit hesitant to let him help me move.

But I did. I could tell when my father saw the infrared sauna, all the shit I had for my Lyme, and one of my rashes, that he realized how serious my condition was. I think he might have thought it wasn't as grave as I was making it out to be. He saw me doing my routine and all the stuff I committed to each and every day, the coffee enema setup, the infrared sauna, the kombucha, and kefir I made on the counter. Something clicked inside him.

Sometimes, I felt uncomfortable with my family because I didn't think they really loved me that much. Now, my father—who had lost his firstborn, Nathan—was witnessing yet another son with a severe health problem. I think something clicked in his brain in that moment, that he may lose another son. He made an effort to connect with me. We began talking more. This was new. Our relationship strengthened instead of the two of us feeling like acquaintances. Some good results do come out of hardships.

My new rush at having my own apartment wore off fast. I hadn't lived alone in a long time, and I'm an extrovert. Plus, I didn't own any furniture to make it inviting for anyone else to come over.

I texted my brother, "I'm living in Utah again," I wrote. "Super crazy with the Lyme and all the coinfections. Who knows what could happen to me. Whether good or bad, either way, I really love you. You mean a lot to me. We should connect while I'm here."

He didn't text back.

My family members and I didn't dislike each other, but we weren't there for each other. I don't think it was purposeful, but more a case of not wanting to deal with the negative emotions ourselves. After Nathan died, I felt like we shut down. Maybe my current Lyme situation was triggering, and nobody wanted to relive that someone-is-severely-sick-in-the-family trauma again. Realizing that my brother wasn't there for me, as I kept waiting for a text that didn't come, was kind of shocking. I thought unconditional love was something families did for each other. I felt like a soldier in a trench who called for backup, and nobody came.

It was hard. It was hard to be rejected like that. The way I saw it, I was coming across as someone who was sick. I was in a dark place. After Nathan's death, they didn't want to handle that. I realized I was going to have to fight this out on my own.

I'm not angry about it now—I know my brother was going through his own struggles. But your psyche takes a certain hit when you are at a dire moment and get ignored.

* * *

I know this much about myself: if I am alone for a day and a half, I go really crazy. After three-plus days, a deep depression sets in. Add in Lyme and all the other random coinfections that mess with your head, and I began losing my mind in that apartment.

People might even call me to go out, but I'd turn them down. I knew I couldn't go to a restaurant or have a drink because I had so many restrictions. I knew I didn't want to have to explain myself to people who would think I was weird. I didn't want to deal with that. I knew I couldn't exercise. So I just got depressed.

To get myself through the day and to make up for the silence, I talked to myself. It's weird when you are that lonely because you think you are making noises out of boredom when really you are talking to yourself because you are fucking lonely.

The only way I can describe the loneliness is that this period of my life was when Taylor and TJ really got to know each other. There was no one else except the two of us and no other choice but to try to understand the deepest parts of myself. On some days, I was so alone and in such pure suffering that I'd just tell myself, *It's TJ and Taylor today*—almost like it was a mantra.

I knew that because of my condition I couldn't produce the way I wanted to produce in work, which really threatened my sense of self-worth. My identity was based on activity and achievement. I had to look hard at the question of, "Who am I if that gets taken away? Can I even love myself if I don't have that?"

You might read that and think, wow, that's messed up. But it was all I knew. No one guided me. No one told me to get good grades. No one told me how to be or what to do. I had no rules after a certain age, and I sort of had to figure out consequences for myself.

I had to parent myself, and I had to figure out how to do that all on my own, while I was down and out with Lyme. Taylor and TJ were how I did it.

Sometimes Taylor would tell TJ, "Yeah, yeah, I love you." And sometimes they'd have a conversation about whether life was going to be worth living if it was going to stay like this. That's when I really had to lean hard on Taylor and my determination to be a friend to myself. "Am I really here for myself?" TJ would ask. "Do I love myself?"

"Let's keep going, man," Taylor would say. "Let's keep going."

As part of trying to take control of my Lyme recovery after the San Diego Police Department picked me up, I stopped working with Dr. Casey. Because my reaction to the doxycycline he had recommended for two weeks was so bad, I'd nearly killed myself and ended up at a psychiatric hospital.

I shared with Dr. Mortell in Utah about the antibiotic cocktail that helped Kurt, the guy with the Lyme success story, and Kurt's Maryland doctor's ideas on how to treat Lyme and coinfections. Even though my experience with doxycycline had been brutal, I thought, "OK, I can rethink my mistrust of antibiotics." Dr. Mortell was willing to work with me so we could alter the protocol together. This new doctor's confidence was invigorating and gave me hope.

At my suggestion, he ordered Coartem, which was developed to treat malaria, and rifampin, an antibiotic used against several types of bacterial infections, which together took away a chunk of my brain fog. There was a certain shade of brain fogginess that never returned after that. I still had brain fog, but it wasn't as bad, like it was a different flavor of fog. This was a win. The protocol didn't wipe me out the way doxy had, and I actually improved.

Then, as the excitement and optimism over the new protocol grew, my grandfather died.

He had been battling cancer and had wanted to pass for a long time. When I really started suffering from Lyme, I understood why my grandfather felt that way. I was so exhausted and tired, with nothing in me, that I got how old people felt, especially if they were fighting something like cancer. Death would be like your friend offering you tickets to go to the beach after you had worked really hard. You could see the beach as an escape, an oasis, relaxation, and a break from the turmoil. When you are that sick, when you are that old, the grim reaper isn't so scary anymore. He isn't trying to violently annihilate you. No, he is offering you a vacation to the beach.

I longed for that beach...that holiday that death could offer...but there was still something inside me that didn't want to quit, the survivor that kept on surviving.

CHAPTER
10

"The worst days are when you feel foggy in the head—chemo-brain, they call it. It's awful because you feel boring. As well as bored. And stupid. And resigned."

—CHRISTOPHER HITCHENS

DR. MORTELL, THE NEW DOCTOR I STARTED WORKING with in Utah, added a regimen of receiving ozone IVs twice a week and intravenous light therapy, also known as IV UV. As I sat there with a needle stuck in my arm, a machine shone various wavelengths of light into my vein. You could see the light inside my skin, which made for a lot of cool Snapchat and Facebook story videos. Then I would do the ozone IV. For the ozone IV, the person administering it would place the bag on the ground before filling it with my blood to a certain level, injecting it with ozone syringes, and letting the blood flow back into me.

These treatments were expensive, so I wrote to the clinic, offering that if I became successful, I would write reviews and publish online about my success. I explained that I was the ideal patient with my organization and proactiveness. They did, indeed, give me a discount.

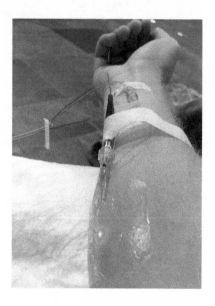

I went to the clinic twice a week, spending four and a half hours there for each IV session. All sorts of patients came in with different ailments, and I was deeply curious about each one. Every person suffering was an instant friend; those with another ailment, like Lupus, for example, became a curiosity.

One guy had such bad Lyme he could only sit in the gravity chair at a certain angle because any pressure on his body hurt like hell. He was so screwed that he had to be in a gravity chair all day—but even that was painful. Anything other than sitting in that chair was excruciating. Although my Lyme was bad, I saw that other people had it way, way worse. Learning this affected me deeply.

The ozone IV cost $450 each time I got it. It gave me relief for a couple of days, but I couldn't tell if the IV UV made a difference or not. No matter, it couldn't hurt.

This was all adding up, and I was feeling the squeeze. My website Dominate Depression was bringing in only a little bit of income, so my friend Jeff, like the saint that he is, helped me buy products off Amazon and eBay and sell them locally on Facebook Marketplace and Craigslist. I made anywhere from twenty-five to fifty dollars in profit per item.

The front desk ladies at my apartment loved me. They didn't care that massive boxes arrived for me regularly (although I think the UPS delivery driver resented me). I would go downstairs, get the items on a dolly, and wheel them up to my room. When someone came to buy them off my ads, I carried them down and sold them for cash. What blew my mind was how few people even opened the boxes and looked at them. It bugged me so much that I would try to get the buyer to look in the box so they could see that I wasn't screwing them over. I'd say, "Are you sure you don't want to check inside?" They'd just shrug. "No, we trust you."

Damn, Utah, you're awesome, but trippy too.

I also was making enough money from buying and selling cryptocurrency to allow me to put some cash aside. Jeff set me up with that gig too. People from all over the country paid me fifty dollars to get on the phone for ten minutes to teach them about cryptocurrency. It was insane. I should have sold it all as the prices rose, because I knew the bubble was going to burst. I watched $8,000 in one account rise to $75,000-plus. I didn't take the advice that I knew I should: "Take the profits where there are profits." Instead of selling, I got greedier and greedier, thinking that I would make it big with a lump sum of money and could use it to cure my Lyme. Emotions tend to blind you like that, and the pain from Lyme did that to me.

* * *

My new Lyme connections in Utah told me about a doctor in Tijuana, Mexico, who injected stem cells into patients—both mesenchymal (from the umbilical cord) and stem cells from sharks. Shark cells might sound off the wall, but they really aren't. Technically, I believe they are "safer" than human ones. There is less of a likelihood of developing issues like Mast Cell Activation Syndrome, which makes you sensitive to everything, including almost all foods, smells, chemicals, and so on. The United States had some weird rules around using stem cells in treatments, dating back to political debates in the early 2000s around abortion and the beginning of life, so I wanted to go to Mexico to get my treatment with the best stuff.

I made the trek all the way over to Tijuana in my 2002 Corolla—stressed out of my mind, sick, and very, very hopeful.

When I finally arrived, I couldn't wait to see the doctor. I greeted people excitedly and spoke Spanish to everybody I came across. I was so optimistic that this clinic could help me.

The clinic ran some blood work, and I explained that Bartonella was my main challenge. The doctors pricked my finger and put my blood under a microscope. After looking at it, they said there were too many Lyme spirochetes and other pathogens in my blood to do a stem cell treatment. These, combined with my antibiotic regimen, would kill the stem cells. There would be no positive effect.

"We can take your money, but we don't recommend it," a doctor told me. Even though this wasn't the news I wanted to hear, I gained a lot of trust in that facility because the doctor was honest with me. I would be back.

Before I left, though, I took up the clinic's suggestion that I try hyperbaric chamber treatments at another office in the same strip mall. A hyperbaric chamber involves breathing pure oxygen while the air pressure in the chamber is raised to a level higher than normal. The increased air pressure helps you absorb more oxygen, which supposedly helps the body heal and fight pathogens. (Pathogens don't like oxygen.)

I had nothing to lose. When I walked in, the salesman at the counter acted like I was the only person he was going to see that day. He was very excited. When I told him I had Lyme, his eyes lit up, but his body language remained the same. He was trying to hide his eagerness—he was certain I represented a paycheck. But his eyes gave it away. He made it seem like the hyperbaric chamber was going to cure me, but I knew he was bullshitting me even though I wanted to believe him.

I got in the chamber and laid down for an hour while wearing an oxygen mask, and he increased the pressure. The experience was relaxing, but I couldn't tell if it helped me.

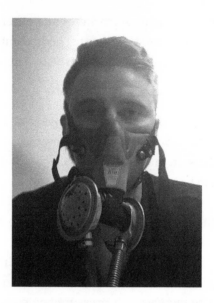

After I got out of the chamber, the salesperson tried to sell me a different device that cost $15,000. In just a few treatments, he said, my Lyme would be cured. This machine would shoot microparticles throughout my body to take the Lyme out. I knew deep down that the method was fake, but again, I wanted to believe him.

Someone who is as sick as I was is one of the easiest people to persuade. At that point, I was so desperate that I listened hard to his pitch and thought about buying the device, even though I knew I wouldn't.

I was devastated that I couldn't get the stem cells. Back down the hope roller coaster again. I headed back to Utah to return to my lonely life, disappointed about the stem cell treatment and unsure if the hyperbaric chamber had helped or not. With all the isolation I was subjecting myself to, my mind wanted to escape more and more. I couldn't take being alone. I couldn't take not being able to focus.

As I drove back home, I called Matt and expressed my frustration. I had driven all that way and not even gotten the stem cells I'd come for.

This big opportunity that could have changed everything for me was a complete waste. My trek was for nothing. But I reminded myself, *At least I tried. At least I was going for it. At least I am attacking Lyme from all angles.*

Next, I tried the ketogenic diet, which basically means eating almost no carbs at all. It was extremely hard, but my brain fog lifted a bit. Even eating too much protein will knock you out of ketosis, so chia seeds in coconut milk started to get old. I stuck to it for two months, then transitioned to a low-carb diet. Although *actual* keto would be incredibly hard to do for extended durations, doing it for a short time helped me.

The brain fog decreased and stayed at a lower level long-term.

* * *

With my high hopes staked on crypto (it hadn't crashed yet), my positivity overflowed onto people. Everyone loved me, including the guy who administered my IV—a little too much. Rodnick was bisexual and always hit on me. I couldn't tell if he was serious, but I started to think he was when he kept mentioning how he wanted to touch my dick a little too much.

It all started one day when I was going over my Lyme symptoms and made the mistake of telling him that I couldn't get an erection anymore because of how sick I was. After that, at every appointment, he asked me how it was going. He told me if it was up to him, he could get it to work. Everyone is a little gay, he said. I assured him I was 100 percent straight. Understand, I don't have a problem with the spectrum or anyone being gay. If I was bisexual, I reassured him, I would be all for it, but I wasn't, and I wasn't interested.

He kept hitting on me and started giving me IVs for free, which saved me hundreds of dollars at a time when money was tight. The whole situation was bizarre and uncomfortable, but I was conflicted. I needed to save money. Looking back, I know the stuff he was saying was downright inappropriate and unhealthy. But I was sick back then and couldn't see the truth of the matter.

During one appointment, I asked him about the ketamine therapy the clinic offered. Ketamine is sometimes used to treat otherwise untreatable depression, anxiety, and PTSD. Turns out it was expensive, and I had to do it under the watchful eye of a therapist.

Rodnick offered to give me a little bit for free, just to try it out. I'd done a lot of drugs back in high school and thought it couldn't be that different of a trip compared to mushrooms and couldn't be worse than salvia.

He injected some ketamine into the side port of the vitamin IV I already had running. After ten seconds, I said, "I don't feel anythhhhh..." and then I was GONE. Instantly the world made a shuddering sound. My vision spiraled downward and to the left in stop-motion, colors changed, and I had no idea what was going on. My body was hard to move, and my head dropped to the side. Then I was in an ambulance.

Holy shit, something happened with the IV. I'm on my way to the emergency room.

The medics in the ambulance were stressed but trying to pretend like they weren't. I was strapped down like an object, unable to move. I started contemplating that this was the end, then realized I had taken ketamine, given to me by someone who wanted to touch my dick.

I opened my eyes and twitched like people were coming for me. I wasn't in an ambulance. I was still in the IV room. I saw Rodnick watching me. He said, "Whoa...whoa, take it easy..." But I didn't trust him.

As he checked my vitals he looked concerned. That scared me even more. He reassured me that I was fine, but I was still freaked. How the hell would I know what he could do to me in this state? I tried to calm down and closed my eyes but could only see all the rape victims in the world. The sensation of being raped ran through me (without it actually happening). I realized how dirty it made me feel and could imagine the feeling of being a victim, how it changes how people see themselves, and their self-image and self-worth afterward. I became deeply sad. Then that image morphed to show all the Lyme victims in the world and their suffering. I saw once again how some people had it way worse than me.

I started crying, and as the tears rolled down my face, I could feel Rodnick shaking me, trying to calm me down, urging, "Please stop. Other people might see you." I saw the fear in his eyes. He didn't want other people to realize I had taken ketamine. I murmured, "They need help, man. They need my help. I gotta help them. I *need* to help them."

"OK, OK, I get it," he whispered, "but please be quiet and stop crying. Just close your eyes and sleep."

Eventually the ketamine wore off enough that I could leave. Rodnick was still really worried he was going to be found out. I let him know I could drive, and he asked in the most concerned tone I had ever heard him use, "Are you *sure*?"

"Yeah, I'm good. Also, don't *ever* give that to me again," I said, like a person who had gone on a roller coaster ride while simultaneously seeing something they can't unsee.

I made it to my car and started sobbing again. Then I called my mother, who I hadn't talked to in a while. I'm not sure why I did; I just felt a strong desire to do so. When I hung up, I sat in my car a bit longer until I knew I could drive, then headed home.

I would definitely not be doing that again anytime soon. I had enough shit to deal with.

CHAPTER
11

"We tend to take a great deal for granted, because you feel like you're going to live forever. It's only if you lose a friend, or maybe have a near-death experience, [that] many events and people in your life suddenly attain real significance."

—BRANDON LEE

ONCE I'D STABILIZED AFTER THE KETAMINE INCIDENT, I started the round of Coartem Dr. Mortell prescribed. Although I took it for two weeks straight—a big no-no for your organs—it was one of the best treatment choices I'd made up to that point. A certain level of brain fog lifted. I still had brain fuzziness, but I could think much clearer. The improvement was like going from driving through the fog and barely being able to see beyond the hood to being able to see ten feet in front of the car. You still can't really see, but at least you can see *something.*

I hope I don't have any permanent damage from aggressive dosing. But I do think the Coartem must have knocked out one of the infections, maybe Babesia. There was a huge change in my body. Sure, I was still sick, but I was a little less sick and a little bit closer to my one dream of being healthy again.

Or so I thought...

My ongoing human guinea pig experiments continued. I tried other antibiotics, including rifampin and clarithromycin. I even tried doxycycline again, although it scared me. The last time I took it, Joseph Smith showed up at my house with handcuffs, so you can understand my hesitancy.

The antibiotics were like flamethrowers to all my gut flora—like doing a microdose of chemo. The antibiotics had as much potential to damage my body as the pathogens did, but if I protected my gut flora it would be a net gain.

I went to a raw dairy farm to get raw goat milk. I made homemade kefir. As I took the antibiotics, I did everything possible to prevent my stomach from getting wrecked. I ate sauerkraut and kombucha. I took probiotics and prebiotics and ate as healthily as possible, slashing my carbs. I was spending virtually my entire life doing supplement preparations and eating and drinking fermented foods.

I was still getting ozone IVs a couple times a week at $450 a session. All these treatments were adding up. In some instances, I spent $1,200 in one day. Many times, I spent over $2,000 in one week. One day, sitting in the chair, I wondered if I could just give myself the IVs. I got the name and model number of the machine the clinic used. Then I joined a Facebook group dedicated to ozone treatments and asked everyone in there about doing the IVs themselves. I learned that most people did ozone rectally or through DIV—meaning you inject the gas straight into your vein. When I asked about the possibility of an embolism happening, I learned that embolisms are rare and only happen when the IVs contain air, which has nitrogen in it. If you are injecting pure ozone and oxygen, an embolism won't happen, since these elements are quickly absorbed into the blood.

I ordered the EXT50 model ozone machine from Longevity; bought a regulator, glass syringe, and needles from eBay; and purchased an oxygen tank from a welding supply company. Oxygen is extremely cheap. I didn't need a medical-grade oxygen tank and prescription, and the oxygen I received at the welding supply shop was exactly the same as what I would get from a medical company. (Remember, I am not giving you medical advice. Whatever you do is at your own risk. I am not responsible if you hurt yourself by trying anything I talk about in this book!)

Since I had already done coffee enemas, I felt comfortable doing a bunch of rectal ozone. But the rectal ozone didn't work that well. I consulted the group again and learned that injecting ozone into my vein is the best way to go. I paid someone in Germany eighty dollars to teach me how to do it over Skype.

One night, I got my whole setup ready to inject ozone DIV-style. People reassured me that this delivery system was normal. They said they never hurt themselves doing it. (However, one of my friends with Lyme told me he used to do it all the time and did it for other people. One girl who came over to have him inject her had a seizure after doing it. No matter; I decided to still take my chances.)

When the big day came for me to administer it to myself, I was nervous. I got everything set up and filled the syringe with ozone, which has the most unique scent of anything I've ever smelled. Then I tried sticking myself, using my left hand, and going into my right arm, but I messed it up. My forearm vein was nice and big, so I went for that instead. When I saw the blood flowing back into the catheter, I knew I'd finally hit it right! *Hell yeah!*

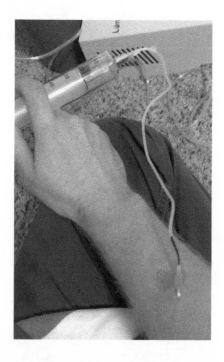

I didn't have medical tape, so I used duct tape to tape the needle down so it would stay in place.

It was time for my moment of truth.

I sat cross-legged on the carpet in my room. The only items around me were my bed and sauna. I had a flash of clarity then of how depressing my existence was, of how I didn't have anything in my house but the raw essentials. I knew I was completely alone; it was just TJ and Taylor at that moment. I was staring at my blood slowly backfilling the catheter, knowing I had to push the syringe to push it back into my body. Nobody else knew what I was doing. It was so risky. This is what my life had become: injecting gas straight into my arm all by myself, hoping it worked out but fully accepting that it might not and being OK with that.

I didn't know if I was doing anything correctly or if I even had the regulator from the oxygen supply set right. And I was a bit sweaty, so it was hard to get the duct tape to stick to my arm.

I took the glass syringe that was loaded up with 50 cubic centimeters of ozone and prepared to inject incremental pushes, having no idea if what I was about to plunge into my arm would permanently maim or kill me. With my left hand on the syringe, I was ready to slowly push 5 ccs at a time into my vein in thirty-second increments. Then I realized I didn't care if I died. Lyme was so shitty it was worth the risk.

Imagine you are in a pure nightmare hell with Satan torturing you. You are witnessing horrible pain and suffering all around you when someone says, "If you try this tactic, you have a chance of getting out of this place. But...there's also a 3 to 5 percent risk that it could make you worse." You'd say yes too— just like I did.

Even if there was a 3 to 5 percent chance of death, I was OK with it if it was my ticket out of hell. I pushed in the plunger and immediately heard a bubbling sound in my vein.

Holy shit, this is wild!

I was sweating from nervousness, but I put the whole dose slowly in my vein anyway. It took longer than I thought to wait thirty seconds in between each push. My lungs felt weird. I started coughing a bit and had to lie down. After lying down for a while, out of it, I felt better. My symptoms improved. I felt a boost in energy, a little less fatigue, and a little less brain fog. I could think more clearly.

Nice!

Once I got the procedure down the right way, I stopped doing ozone IVs at the clinic for the most part—and I made my money back on the machine within a week and a half. That was one of the fastest returns on any investment I'd ever made in my life.

Once I was in a routine of doing the ozone injections at home, I encountered a new problem: increased depression from loneliness.

When I was getting IVs at the clinic, I hung out with people like me for eight hours a week. After I learned to dose myself, I sometimes did an IV at the clinic simply because I wanted to be back in that room. I was paying money to avoid loneliness. I wanted to be back talking to people who understood and knew me. I wanted to escape the loneliness of just TJ and Taylor hanging out together.

* * *

Because I was taking so many antibiotics, I was getting some new strange symptoms. At one point, my left eye started randomly twitching from all the medications I was on. It was extremely annoying because my brain couldn't filter it out.

After you have Lyme for a while, so many whacked-out symptoms occur in your body that they don't phase you. It's just one traumatizing symptom or experience after another. You get used to it.

You get weird symptoms that would freak someone else out to the point they'd need therapy for a month to get over it, but you take it in stride. When you're chronically ill, it's just another day. You become numb to how bizarre it is for your body to act up. You only briefly remember how serious your situation is.

One day while I was lying in bed, at about 2:00 p.m. in the middle of the week, suddenly something in my body felt off. My body felt heavier than normal—like when you wake up in the middle of a dream, and you think you can't move a muscle.

As I lay there, the heaviness crept up toward my head. Then, I tried to move, and I *couldn't*. White light filled in the outer edge of my vision. I lost sight of the infrared sauna on the right side of my bed in my little room until white light was all I could see, and all my pain suddenly went away.

I saw my dead brother, my dead best friend, and my dead grandfather come to me.

Wow...this is it. Sometimes you just randomly...die.

It was warm, and my constant suffering was coming to an end. I wasn't scared but felt more of a final relief and escape from my chronic and silent suffering.

It's finally over. This is what it must feel like to be old and tired and ready to die. Now it's my turn.

I don't know how much time passed, but when I came to, my body was still so heavy I couldn't move. But I was so out of it. I didn't have thoughts, and I couldn't process what was going on. Everything was calm. At peace. Then my mind slowly came back. I was terrified, paralyzed. *Maybe that's what people feel like when they are still conscious during surgery.*

My only working body part was my eyelids. I stared at my ceiling. Then I went out again.

I came to two more times, each time having the same experience. Then at 5:00 or 6:00 p.m., I started coming to for real. The heaviness dissipated as I returned to life. I stared down at my body, which wanted to move. Finally, I could flex my hands, then my arms. I twisted my wrists back and forth. It took a few minutes before I could move the rest of my body. When I could, I sat up and absorbed the moment.

Hoooooly shit. What was that...?

The experience was humbling. I'd completely lost control. I couldn't do anything when Lyme made me its bitch. It was going to do with me what it wanted in that moment. I didn't have a choice in the matter. I think we all forget that we could lose control at any time, and there's nothing we can do when that happens.

I'd gone in and out of consciousness for three hours or more. It wouldn't have mattered if someone had tried to call me, and it would have been impossible for me to have called for help. I couldn't have dialed 911.

I would have just laid there, no matter the outcome. Nobody would have known.

This was a Taylor and TJ experience. I couldn't just go around sharing my experience with other people. That moment had to be locked away, categorized as another bizarre Lyme experience out of the hundred that had affected me. It was too heavy for others. People don't want to deal with that level of darkness. I had to deal with it all by myself.

* * *

No matter what happened, I had to keep moving forward and push my fear to the side. Even though trauma can take a piece of your optimistic soul, I had no other choice but to carry on.

Well...I actually did have another choice, and I knew it.

I wrote in my journal, "I think if I can't figure out the health stuff in a year or so, it'll be time to join that place." Giving my brain that "out" relieved pressure even if after a year, I'd rewrite my decision: "OK, one more year and then if I'm still sick, I'll let myself die." It just felt easier to continue on if there was an end date in sight. I was bargaining with my brain with suicide carrots. It wanted it to be over, but I ordered my mind to give it just a bit more time to see if anything turned around, dangling the carrot just a little bit further in the future to keep me going.

You might be reading this and thinking, *Of course, you could have shared that with people, TJ! You don't have to go through that alone!*

Wrong.

You can only share a little bit. I was in hell every single day. If I'd expressed how bad it was, it would be *too dark*.

Other people can't take on that level of misery and darkness all the time—they have their own lives to live. I didn't want to become an obligation to them. That's why I've always tried my best to joke around and be positive around others, to try to keep it light at times—because I had already lost my entire life and most of the people around me. I didn't want to lose the people who were still there by pulling them down into hell with me.

I compare this to the same reason we might not feel that bad when we walk by homeless people on the street, people with missing limbs, parents with skinny, dying kids, or those who ask for money for their limping dog. The suffering is all around us, but you have to ignore it at some level. If you let all the darkness of the world in, it will consume you.

What I was living was a dark, heavy, walking hell. I had to shield that from people—even if inside, my brain was begging me to end the suffering. Other people didn't see that because I shared it rarely and only with certain people. I was most grateful for the people who stuck around even after experiencing the weighty hell that was my life.

CHAPTER
12

"Your only path to success is through a continuum of mundane, unsexy, unexciting, and sometimes difficult daily disciplines compounded over time."

—DARREN HARDY

MORE TESTING SHOWED THAT MY HORMONES WERE OFF. If your hormones are off, it's very hard to get better from Lyme, if not impossible, according to the doctor. Therefore, Dr. Mortell put me on thyroid and testosterone medicines.

My testosterone was around three hundred—in the range of someone over sixty years old. Your thyroid affects many, many hormones. If your thyroid is messed up that can cause anxiety, fatigue, muscle weakness, and weight problems.

The doctor offered to inject a pebble into my ass cheek that would slowly release testosterone. He said I could also inject it intramuscularly. I opted for the intramuscular syringe. The testosterone seemed a little risky because, long-term, my body could become dependent on it, and then I would have to take it the rest of my life. It could mess up my ability to have kids. I started off injecting about 0.5 mL twice a week, which at 200 mg/mL, was 100 mg twice per week.

After the first injection, I got a burst of energy, so I knew it was working. I didn't think the hormones were going to fix everything about Lyme, but it seemed they could help a lot with some of the problems I was dealing with.

It felt great to have that creative, generative, sexual energy back. It was so central to who I was and to everything I wanted to do in my life.

After a couple of weeks, my body was saturated with testosterone.

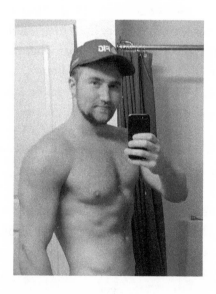

I went from 183 pounds to 197 in a little over a month or two with minimal body fat gain while lightly lifting weights. I was excited. Understandably, I thought I was getting better! But once again I forgot to stay humble and keep my feet on the ground. I was too excited—which meant I didn't see the fall coming.

I was so confident that the testosterone was working on my Lyme disease that I called Matt and exclaimed, "It's my hormones, bro! I should be able to start working and getting shit done again." He was excited about it also. My libido was so high that a couple of times, when I saw an attractive woman walking down the street, I pulled over and got her phone number. Yes, it was a little manic, but damn, it was nice feeling whole again. That beautiful part of life had been taken away from me.

However, the testosterone shrank my balls. I was nervous it could cause them to atrophy permanently, but the doctor assured me it wasn't a big deal. And after being on the testosterone regimen for a while, my Lyme flared up. Even though I was still on testosterone, it wasn't having that positive effect any longer. I started to feel shitty again.

It was the hope roller coaster again, from hurt to better and back to square one. There was no doubt in my mind; I was still messed up. Not only that, but it turned out I'd been taking way too much testosterone. A check showed my levels had jumped from 380 to almost 2,000—way too high. No wonder I was jumping out of my car to chat up pretty women. That high level was risky if I ever wanted to have kids.

I decreased my testosterone dose and got it closer to the 700–800 range, which is more of a normal range for a twenty-one- to twenty-four-year-old. Yet I still felt like shit.

The next thing I tried was taking my raw DNA from 23andme. com and plugging my results into different apps and other online sites. By doing that I figured out that I have the MTHFR and COMT genetic mutations.

MTHFR (also referred to as motherfucker gene) affects a lot of people with Lyme. That mutation can cause depression, anxiety, and bipolar disorder, since it can lead to high levels of homocysteine and low levels of folate and other B vitamins. I needed to supplement with additional methyl forms of B vitamins to counteract it (which I now know is debatable as to whether that is the best thing to do).

A COMT mutation limits the body's ability to remove catechol (a molecule that includes dopamine, norepinephrine, etc.), so I had to take alpha-lipoic acid and NAC to help. I felt a little improvement from the additional supplements. But significant improvement is a gradual thing. When you are in so much pain, it takes a while to get better, even though you want instant results.

* * *

The pressure is on when you are trying to make new friends. You have to be proactive if you want to be social even if you have Lyme. As a man I felt that when I went on dates, I must lead the way; I must make the plans; I must direct the conversation so the connection could continue.

Lyme symptoms can go up and down, with some weeks much worse than others. Every now and then, I would have some slight relief from Lyme and go on a great date. In these brief reprieves, I would vibe and connect with my date. After two weeks, the wrecking truck would come by and run me over again while I was sleeping. I'd wake up destroyed for the next month. Predictably, the relationship would fade away.

Then I'd go on a new date with a new woman. We would connect, and eventually, I would crash, and the relationship would fade. Rinse and repeat.

Another dating complication is that I can't eat out because I'm sensitive to almost all foods. In any restaurant or bar, I can only order sparkling water. To protect my health, I banned myself from 95 percent of the social activities that people use to bond. It always weirded out a date when I'd take them to a restaurant or bar, and I had already eaten beforehand, or I only consumed water.

Everything was a reminder of how sick I was. Each time I had to say no to the waitress, each time I said I couldn't drink, each time I had to turn down going hiking or some other activity, I was reminded of how sick I was. After so much of this, eventually, you stop putting yourself out there. You don't want the reminders.

One more reason not to date: I couldn't predictably get an erection. My libido was so low I simply couldn't get it up most of the time. Some women would leave me when that happened. Eventually I got a prescription for Viagra, and once in a while, I would take it and have sex simply to give a woman what I knew she wanted. But I didn't really enjoy it. I did it for them.

The Viagra showed me something else; it helped with some of my Lyme symptoms, and I was more clear-headed on it. It turns out I was having blood-flow issues throughout my whole body. This was an example of why it was so important for me to tell my doctors everything, since I didn't know what might be a clue that could guide them.

Most people go to the doctor and think it's up to the doctor to heal or cure them. They put themselves in the doctor's hands. That's wrong, whether you're seeing a physician or a therapist or someone else. The practitioner can help—they might be able to do 20 percent of the work. But you have to do 80 percent. They are going to talk to you for maybe thirty minutes in a busy day. If you just show up passively and wait for them to figure you out, they aren't very likely to do so.

If you're dealing with Lyme, you almost certainly have a long medical history. You can't expect your doctor, who has many patients, to take the time to dig through it. You have to help them help you. You've got to show up for them and make their job easier. They only know what you tell them, so be prepared to tell them the important things. If you keep detailed records of what's happening and what you've been doing about it, they're more likely to find a pattern of clues and be able to work effectively with you. You'll only be helped to the extent that you come prepared to be helped.

I created a folder in Google Drive called "Health History." Every time I get a lab or test result, I convert it into a PDF and name it consistently—a description of the test and the date. An example would be, "2018.4 Hormonal Panel" which would mean in April of 2018 I tested all my hormones. If a doctor wants to know, "When did you last get your thyroid tested?" I can find it in two clicks. So can they, because I share that folder with them and I make it super intuitive for them to navigate it. This makes it extremely easy to work with doctors. Alright, back to my libido.

* * *

Lyme messed with my libido for a long time. Sometimes it wiped it out completely; other times, it took it to extremely low levels. It yo-yoed like that for years. Most people think that libido refers to an animal drive to have sex. But sexual energy is a big sign of vitality. You can use sexual energy in creative ways: to build a business, exercise, write music, etc. Sex drive can be one of the most potent forces that we have access to. Without it, my life was very gray and flat. I was a machine with flesh attached, going through the motions with no real desire or enjoyment of anything.

From around 9:00 a.m. to 4:00 p.m., I did repetitive health tasks, day in and day out, by myself, without fail. This was one of the most mundane experiences of my life, but I knew it was necessary. Lots of people say they "want" success—they want the nice car, they want a million dollars, they want to be healthy—but they are never willing to pay the price. Lyme recovery involves a massive price tag. Sometimes I wondered if I was capable and willing to pay it.

A typical day when I was living in Utah went like this:

- Wake up around 9:00 a.m. (sometimes, I'd lie in bed until noon).

- Take all my supplements and tinctures (these take a while to prepare).

- Meditate in the sun.

- Drink a healthy smoothie with more supplements (this also required lots of prep).

- Do a coffee or ozone enema.

- Go for a forty-five-minute walk.

- Eat a healthy meal (this also took a while to prepare) consisting of every good-for-you ingredient from bison to seasonings to kimchi to homemade raw goat milk kefir (kefir took time to prep and make), with more supplements, at around 12:00 p.m.

- Use a dry skin brush before getting into the infrared sauna for thirty minutes.

- During the sauna session, do sesame oil swishing in my mouth, aka "oil pulling."

- Get in a detox bath for thirty minutes or more with Epsom salts, Himalayan sea salt, apple cider vinegar, hydrogen peroxide, essential oils, tea bags, and baking soda. It would be about 2:30 p.m. by this point.

- Sometimes do an ozone IV (administered myself).

- Try to stretch.

- Review doctor notes, reorder supplements, prepare for the next day, etc.

Finally, I would begin my day at around 4:00 p.m. Later, I would have a super healthy dinner with more supplements, and at night, I would make my special drink and supplements/tinctures.

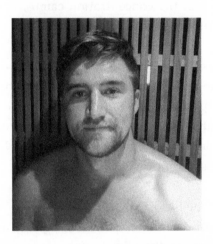

While other people were at work in the office, I was at work on my health and body.

Sometimes I wondered if it was worth it because I wasn't necessarily getting better, and I had lots of ups and downs. It's really hard to stay motivated and positive when you are doing everything in your power to win, and it feels like you are only inching forward.

My choices were to either keep trying or die. If it was all a waste, too bad. But if there was a 2 percent chance I could get better, then it would be worth it. That's how I had to frame it in my mind.

* * *

Viktor Frankl said in his book *The Will to Meaning* that the optimists in the Holocaust always died or committed suicide first. It was the realists who survived. The optimists would say, "We'll be free by Christmas." But then Christmas would pass, and they were still stuck in the concentration camps. Eventually, they couldn't endure the constant letdowns.

I felt like I was battling a similar mindset as I rode the roller coaster of hope and disappointment, of getting better and then relapsing. I kept thinking one treatment was going to work; I would get excited and feel a bit better, only to come crashing down and get depressed. I thought I'd be "better by Christmas," but Santa Claus never came.

If you think of me like a car, before I had Lyme I could go over one hundred miles per hour, hell, I could go 140 miles per hour, but I had to have the discipline to go no more than twenty-five now with Lyme. I had to learn to put my health first. I have struggled and struggled with that.

The hard thing is I know I'm a Lamborghini. I know I can go 140-plus, and I know I'm sticking at twenty-five. Do you know how boring it is to drive a Lamborghini that's stuck at twenty-five miles per hour? Sometimes I just couldn't stand it and I drove 140 anyway, and I'd suffer the consequences. My vehicle, my body, would break and then be in the shop for days at a time to recover. It's hard not to drive that thing the way it's supposed to be driven every now and then.

It was very frustrating. I was angry. I know what I'm capable of. Normally, if I had a business dispute and somebody screwed me over, I'd come back at them hard. But I had to tell myself, "Don't wear yourself out." I had to restrain myself. I felt like an Olympic athlete sidelined with a broken ankle. I knew that if I could play the game I would win, but I couldn't play. People might tell me to "think positive," but no amount of positive thinking gets over a broken ankle, and no amount of positive thinking gets over Lyme.

I have to accept a redefinition of who I am, and I am angry at Lyme for making me do that.

One day, I took Mike Posner's "I Took a Pill in Ibiza," changed the lyrics, and renamed it "I Took Some Antibiotics." I recorded myself playing the song with all my supplements and medical stuff in the background. When I posted it to Facebook, I didn't care who saw it, even though it revealed how hard my life was.

I Took Some Antibiotics

I took some antibiotics...to show the Lyme I know what's up.

Symptoms were all over, and my gut was ten years older but fuck it, I don't know what to do.

I'm living out in Utah.

Infrared sauna in my room.

I'm losing money daily cuz I'm healing like crazy cuz I spend it on ozone tools.

(Chorus)

You don't wanna be sick, like me.

All coming from one tick, like me.

You don't want to be researching every hour, all alone.

You don't want to be tired like this. When you need to sleep wired like this...

You don't ever wanna be stuck up in your home singing...stuck up in your home singing.

Aaaaaaall. I knooow. I've no idea. Which doctor is right or wrong.

Singing aaaalll. I know. I have no idea. When this will be gone.

(End of Chorus)

I'm just a top salesman. Who lost all he had.

I get along with old friends cuz I focus on the trend of making big money once again.

I can't keep a girl, noooo. Always love me at first sight.

But when I crash for three weeks pushing back the next meet, they all think I'm ghosting them upright.

(Chorus)

Had to go back to my hometown. I brought my mindset and my smile.

My friends are still here, but we've aged different years, and they're not sure why I can't run a mile.

I walked around downtown. People eating at McDonald's.

They say you look healthy like a model, so here's a beer bottle, so I looked them in the eyes, and I said...

(Chorus)

Aaaaaaall. I knooow. Is I have no ideaaa. No ideaaaa.

Singing aaaalll. I know. I have no idea. But I won't stop fighting till it's gone.

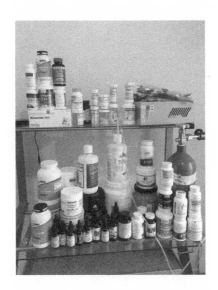

If you want to hear the song, use the QR code below. Just forgive the poor singing skills:

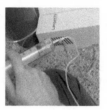

There was something healing about expressing myself in a song. It was like having a ton of suppressed emotions and an inability to communicate with the normal world, then letting it rip and saying, "Fuck it! I'm putting that message out there."

Around that time, I found a support group for Lyme in Utah. It was one of the best support groups ever. The organizer, Danielle, had a huge heart. One day when my Bartonella was flaring I decided I would bring my guitar and sing my song to the group. On one hand, I had extreme anxiety, but Bartonella also caused such intense mood swings that other times I had the confidence of someone given a mission delivered directly from God.

While I was driving there, I felt like God was telling me to share my song. I was a bit insecure about performing, but I kept hearing a message in my head: *It's not about you; it's about them.* Besides, I knew from doing improv and stand-up that when it came to public speaking or playing a song in front of people, stage fright means I need to put the focus on them. If I directed my focus onto others, I tended to forget about myself. My anxieties and worries didn't matter so much.

There were eight people present, and I think they were surprised that I was actually going to play and sing. When I started to play, I could see their defensive walls drop a little bit. A few of them even teared up. I could feel their emotion, and they could feel mine. When I finished, they thanked me. It was a quick journey from skepticism on their part and nervousness on mine to gratitude on their part and a sense of being seen and accepted on mine.

I felt invigorated doing something so vulnerable and feeling seen for it. It's so hard to share the reality of Lyme with people who can't understand what you're going through. But these people could because they were going through it too.

CHAPTER
13

"Courage is not having the strength to go on; it is going on when you don't have the strength."

—TEDDY ROOSEVELT

BY THE MIDDLE OF 2018, AFTER EIGHT MONTHS IN UTAH, I was running out of money. My online pursuits were only bringing in around $4,000 per month, and with my medical expenses that wasn't enough.

I had saved up enough money when I was selling solar door-to-door in Texas to last me this long, but times were difficult. One of my friends in Arizona, Jake, was selling solar in Phoenix. He told me that I could make selling easier on myself if I moved there and worked in his company because I could run their pre-set appointments without knocking doors.

I knew I had to bust a move, and I liked this plan. I found and rented an apartment in Arizona, but after driving all the way down with my friend Jonny who joined me on the journey to help, when I got to Tempe and opened the apartment door it was incredibly dusty and reeked of chemical cleaners. Every part of my body flared, and my inflammation was off the charts. I thought I was having a complete breakdown. I felt as if my brain was dissolving away, like what happens when gas is poured on Styrofoam.

I couldn't possibly move in with those toxic smells and dust. My head spun, causing dark pain. It was so bad I wanted it all to end. Again. I moved out to a hotel. After enough time and enough cleaning, I moved in. I was still paranoid that the apartment had chemicals all over it and a ton of dust was still on the blinds, in the crevices, and elsewhere. My mother flew down to help me clean up the apartment since there was still dust everywhere. I had to make sure it wasn't going to destroy me.

Despite that incident, I liked the feeling of Arizona a lot. People were chill, it was hot (I don't like the cold or darkness), and Scottsdale was fun to visit and near my apartment in Tempe. Phoenix was massive, so I assumed it had a lot of potential.

After coming out of my Lyme flare from the apartment, I was ready to start my new job and get back into solar sales. It felt awesome to return to what I knew. This company knew about my health issues, and I didn't have to be knocking doors to set up appointments anymore. My new team only had a couple of people. Back in my SolarCity days, if someone was ahead of me in sales, I lost sleep over it until I was ahead of them again. Now, I needed to work in a company where my competitive drive wouldn't push me beyond my health limits. This was the best fit. I knew if I had taken a job working for a big name brand or any other solar company, I'd collapse from pushing myself too hard because my ego wouldn't protect me—I wouldn't be able to stand losing.

But reality slapped me in the face when I started going to people's homes and selling again. I wasn't as good at closing as I used to be because I was so tired and out of it. I didn't have my usual charisma. I lacked energy. People didn't like me because I came across as a tired, weird dude. Lyme forced me to pivot again. I had to learn to sell people on pure strategy and tactics alone—I couldn't rely on them being sold on *me* anymore.

Even though I didn't need to, I still went out knocking just to get into the field and earn some sales. But I always got tired and couldn't finish what I started.

That made me sad. Back in the day, I used to get invited to clients' family parties, to weddings, and to eat dinner with them. Now, I could no longer accept any food offered to me.

I used to be a hardcore rep, able to break through any mental barrier and knock doors all day. Now, I purposely had to go slow. Lyme had robbed me of another one of my core identities.

But not entirely. Sometimes I still summoned the old TJ magic.

One day, I knocked on a guy's door in Tempe just west of my apartment on McClintock Road. He swung the door open, saw me, and immediately shut it in my face. Right after he shut it, I re-knocked the door, and he yanked it open and angrily asked what I wanted. I hit him with my pitch, and he asked if I needed to get into his attic. The next thing I knew, his garage door was opening. Within a few minutes, I was inside his attic.

When I left, he said, "Don't come back if it costs more than $5,000." When I returned, the guy said his daughter would take over the home eventually. I scheduled a time on another day where all of us could sit together. On that day, I showed up with my manager, Jake, and we quoted the guy and his daughter $21,000; he put $5,000 down and signed the agreement.

At another appointment in Arizona City, I was the fifteenth solar person to sit down with the homeowner. In the end, he hit me with the dreaded "I need to think about it" line, which meant I'd screwed up somewhere in the sales process. He wouldn't budge. I asked what he needed to research and how long that would take. He said, "Until next year in the month of June." I told him, "If it doesn't make sense now, it won't make sense in a year."

I left assuming it was a lost cause. There's probably only a 5 percent chance in solar after presenting and leaving a homeowner's house that it will lead to a sale later.

But I was wrong. The homeowner called me up and had more questions. At the end of the call, he asked, "When can you get here?"

When I showed up, he was still not sold. He just kept hitting me with questions and getting lost in his analysis. He led me into his kitchen, where we took seats at the table while Michael Jackson played in the background. As I sat there with him, I got that sinking feeling. *I drove all the way out here for nothing.* Then out of nowhere with desperation kicking in, I got up and busted into a side glide and moonwalk in his kitchen. He laughed, and when I sat back down I said, "Look, you've spent lots of time on this already. You know I am the best option, and you'll only be wasting more time putting this off further. Let's just get this process started, alright?" I called that my moonwalk close.

I even closed a guy who threatened to kill me every time I showed up at his house in Maricopa. He told me that if he did kill me, it would look like I had died a natural death at a family party with a lot of witnesses. That way, nobody would know I had been poisoned or murdered. One time, I showed up at his house and he had a big gun pointed at the entryway to try to scare me.

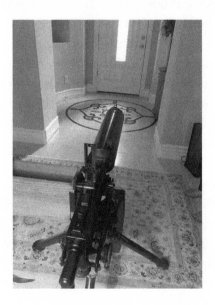

Those moments of brief bouts of energy reminded me of what I used to be able to do. They were glimpses into my past. Without energy, you can't even think of getting up and breaking into a moonwalk to get a prospect to close.

That's what I love about sales. It takes complete confidence in yourself to be good at it, and you never know what to expect.

Most days, however, were not anywhere near that good.

One time my manager came with me to an appointment I ran while I was super sick. He was shocked at how shitty I did. I knew I couldn't blame it on the Lyme, even though that was the problem. Instead, I took the feedback. Driving home, I was depressed. I could have gotten the deal if I weren't sick, but I *was*. Sometimes I didn't know how to carry on.

The hardest part was how shitty I felt while trying to do this, all alone in the chemical apartment by myself. It got to the point again where I legitimately wanted to die on a regular basis. I wore my Carlos necklace every single day. Every morning, in pure hell and agony, I would grab the dog tag, think about my friend, and tell myself I would continue. It was almost like if I committed suicide, it would be an insult to *his* suicide. With that thought banging around my head, I would go to my first appointment of the day.

After that appointment, I would drive back to my apartment, lie in my bed until the next appointment, then grab onto Carlos's dog tag. As I grasped it, I would try to reach my higher spiritual self—the self that went beyond my waning energy. I would force myself to get up, hit the next appointment, then come home to lie down again.

Day after day, I did this, barely making it to my sales appointments. When I arrived at an appointment, right before I walked in, I felt like a soldier on his last leg of exhaustion—ready to die.

As I walked up to the door, I'd pump myself up: *all you have to do is give it your all for an hour and a half, then you can lie down again.*

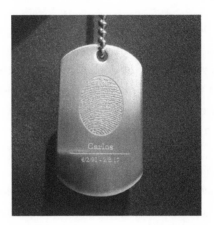

Every day, I wished I was dead, but for some reason, I didn't die.

While I fought all these frightening urges, I poured out my problems to a couple of friends on the phone. One friend, Arielle, asked me to open up to her. I told her I didn't trust becoming vulnerable because I had been abandoned and left behind before, and it was too painful to risk that again. I was still fighting the pain I experienced when people left me because of the Lyme. Arielle assured me that she would never leave me. Yet as we talked, as I let her into my nightmare, she drifted away, stopped responding, then ghosted me for two months.

That hurt. In my head, I was so broken that even a person who had promised not to leave me couldn't handle it and left anyway.

I have a different perspective on the situation now. I'm not mad. I understand. What I was going through was way too heavy for anyone to take on all the time. But in the moment, it's painful in the realization of how messed up you really are.

Now, I see the loss of those friends as something that made me stronger. It reinforced my ability to be self-sufficient and survive through unnerving pain. I dug deep to move past the despair that made me want to blow my head off. I got strong enough to look that pain in the eyes and continue another day. There was no point in being a victim. Taylor and TJ had to prevail.

I was forced to create meaning out of that experience. Was it a good experience? No, but it happened. I got to ask myself what I was going to do with it. Experiences like this taught me that people turn away from someone with Lyme. Lyme disease is a heavy burden. Why would someone choose to take that on if they don't have to? A lot of people can't handle it if you try to lean on them. They're not strong enough to take that darkness or weight. I don't blame them.

I knew I had to keep moving forward regardless. If I had support? It would make it easier. But if I didn't? I had to keep going anyway.

CHAPTER
14

"Rock bottom will teach you lessons that mountaintops never will."

—UNKNOWN

No matter the meds I was on or the treatments I tried, the extreme ups and downs were relentless.

In mid-September of 2018, I was hit with a harsh relapse and my hand broke out in a massive rash.

It progressed to looking abnormal, and people could see it, so they asked about it.

"That's the Lyme flaring up." I didn't know exactly what was causing it. Maybe Bartonella, maybe something else. When you have Lyme you have coinfections, and of course, I was battling several different tick-borne diseases.

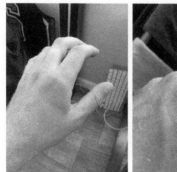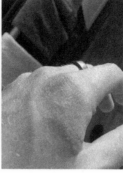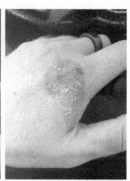

Their faces would contort in confusion, and they'd say, "Lyme does that?"

"Yep." I'd shrug.

"Weird..."

It was one of the few times people could actually see evidence of the ways Lyme ravaged me.

To me, that rash was a confirmation of how bad my flare-up was. I was afraid that I was spiraling, unsure of how bad it was about to get.

I was lonely, sick as hell, and once again fighting my demons. I slogged through monotonous days of waking up, going to an appointment, and coming back to lie in bed, only to have to use some sort of higher power just to get up and go at it again.

One day, it was too much. I sent a couple of texts to some people about how I wasn't doing well, got in my car, started it up, rolled down my windows, and closed my garage.

I was sitting in the running car when my friend Lacy called.

"Hey, how are you?"

"Not very good."

It was one of those moments that makes a big difference in your life. Maybe all the difference. She could hear that something about my answer was off.

"What are you doing?" she asked carefully.

"I'm sitting in my car with it running and the garage door shut."

"Do you want to open the garage door?"

She convinced me to turn the car off. I opened the garage and went back upstairs.

Was I just asking for help, asking to be seen in my suffering? Would I have sat in the car until it was too late? I don't know. Maybe I wouldn't have noticed I was dying because carbon monoxide just puts you to sleep, and the last fear response would have faded away before I could do anything about it.

Maybe I did want to die that day. A lot of times a suicide attempt is a cry for help, and that may be what I was doing. I can't put my finger on it. I only know I was in enough pain to sit in my car for a lengthy period of time while it pumped carbon monoxide into a closed space.

That's scary to think about.

Those are the types of experiences you can't tell people. Well, I guess I'm telling you now. That shit is heavy, and my experience was that when I shared heavy stuff I scared people away. It's hard to understand. It's hard to relate to. It's hard to know how to deal with it.

After that experience, I couldn't sleep. When I have insomnia, that's when songs fly into my head. That's when I don't have inhibitions. I started writing real stuff and not caring what people thought.

Trying to be strong wasn't enough. Expressing the truth helped. And the truth was that no matter how strong I was, I still needed people to help me, but I didn't feel like I had very many I could count on.

This is the song I wrote.

I Was Told...

Effort and mindset, that's all I need.

Don't be upset; your thoughts can mislead.

But you get ill, and your only bet is treatment.

You realize the book The Secret *is just lazy and convenient.*

Suicidal thoughts twenty-seven days out of thirty.

All alone because others getting tired of being worried.

You know it is the illness, but these thoughts are full of stigma.

Suicidal and tired isn't exactly the recipe for charisma.

I was told...

Family will always be there.

Especially if you get lost in a maze of despair.

But back home in Utah, I'm only to discover

I'm still alone in this jigsaw, even ignored by my own brother.

Each day I just know it is TJ and Taylor.

I can't grow when I'm always so near to failure.

Each day, I've learned to come off strong and fun.

But really, I've just lost my concern that I wish my life was done.

I was told...

With effort, my life can be full of wealth.

But not the impossibility of life with no energy or health.

That life will work out, and you just have to find the key.

But not that sometimes we just get slapped by harsh reality.

Life isn't always meant to be simple and easy.

It's not the universe's job to get out of its way to please me.

I always judged older people when they didn't have any joy.

Instead of asking myself, maybe something in their life got destroyed.

I was told...

Everything is possible in life and business.

Nobody showed me chronicles of loss and sickness.

So maybe what we all desperately need,

Is to realize that sometimes as humans, we bleed.

I recorded that song the night I wrote it—May 18, 2018. You can hear it here:

I was learning that performing like this helped. I felt that, on the one hand, I knew I had to be strong and keep pushing forward no matter what. I would try and try, even though I didn't have the support I wanted. I would compartmentalize, I would suppress emotions. But I couldn't keep them in because it wreaked havoc within me. Emotions turned into physical pain. I found that if I told the truth—not to just anybody, but to the right people, people who could get me and see me and hear me—I expelled those emotions. I let that out of my body, which brought relief.

I was able to go from "I can't keep doing this," to "OK, we have our routines, let's do the infrared sauna, let's do the detox, let's keep going a little longer." It was like talking myself through a marathon. I was still using suicide carrots, promising myself I could kill myself if I had to, but I wouldn't just yet.

* * *

Soon, I was at rock bottom again.

In addition to my severe depression, feeling stupid all the time was scary and frustrating. Interacting with people and the world, I knew what I would normally be capable of, but I just couldn't do it. I knew some people saw me as an idiot. I also knew I couldn't do anything to change that perception because my brain fog was that intense.

I went into a gun store in Tempe, but I couldn't buy a pistol because I didn't have an Arizona license. I could only buy a rifle or a shotgun. It didn't seem like an easy way to go, blowing my head off by using my damn toe to pull the trigger. The last thing I wanted to do was mess up.

Matt called while I was in the store, and I told him I couldn't buy a handgun. He asked me why I was trying to buy a gun. But I forgot. I'd driven to the store depressed, but once I got inside the store, I was numb.

The gravity of how sick and bad I felt overwhelmed me. I didn't realize how insane it was that I was trying to buy a gun to keep in my house until I heard the concern in my friend's voice.

Mission aborted, I left the store, got in my car, and started driving aimlessly, crying my eyes out.

"I wish I could understand what you are going through, but I can't. Just know that I am here for you, man," Matt said.

Matt saved me. Just as Lacy had saved me, he was able to be there when I needed it. I was able to talk myself out of eating that suicide carrot. I was able to look at myself and say, "OK, are you really ready to hold a gun to your head and pull the trigger?" And the answer I got back was, "No. Not now."

Matt saying he was there for me was all I needed to hear. He wasn't trying to give me advice. He wasn't telling me that other people have it worse. I didn't need advice. I just needed someone to truly hear me. I needed to be validated. I needed someone to see and understand the prison I lived in.

I let it all out. All the suppressed sadness, fears, despair, worries, and hopelessness. It was all buried inside, and now it came to the surface. I cried for ten minutes on the phone to him, driving aimlessly around Tempe.

Afterward, I wrote this:

It's like being innocent charged with a crime.

Stuck in the cell of my body, passing the time.

Unable to have energy and experience my youth.

Used to fake positive but now I'm telling the truth.

Yeah, of course, I'm scared.

I experience trauma almost every single day of the year.

Feeling like I'm going to break and finally implode.

Any good day without aches is life on easy mode.

Stressed, my body is constantly full of histamine.

Each day I'm foggy, not sure if I'll see the game over screen.

I don't got a church, a community, or place of rest.

On a constant search as Taylor and TJ are put to the test.

* * *

Although my first experience with a Rife machine had left me skeptical, I was hearing from some people in the Lyme Facebook groups that they had experienced good results. I thought,

"Well, maybe it doesn't work. But let's give it a shot. Worst-case scenario, I lose four grand, best-case scenario, I fix my Lyme." I purchased the True Rife.

The machine is a box that can run various programs. I could attach different devices to it—I had a device I could submerge into footbaths, and another device that flashed a light at particular frequencies. The bottoms of your feet are supposedly a high-detox spot, so I would put my feet in a bath with a little salt and water and the device and let it run an ionic foot bath Lyme detox program. I used the bulb in my bed while I slept. I put it right under the covers with me, where it flashed a particular sequence of frequencies that was supposed to help me detox while I slept.

I did feel I got some relief from the footbaths, and I still do them occasionally. I was trying so many things it was hard to tell what was working, but it did seem like it helped.

When women I dated saw the bulb in my bed, they thought it was strange. Who wouldn't? I used it even when I had company. Imagine what the experience was like for a woman who joined me in a bed that contained flashing lights and made slight beeping sounds. Let's just say it didn't help.

Sometimes, I got so sick and was so out of it that my brain felt on *fire*. I felt like all my neurons were blasting away, and the pain sped up to an intense level, making me want to do something, anything, to feel better. In those moments I would bust out the ionic footbath with the Rife machine while simultaneously injecting ozone directly into a vein. The combo dulled the edge. It took me from *Holy shit, I cannot take this anymore and am going to shoot myself* down to the relatively tolerable level of *I cannot take this anymore.*

One night, after I started a regimen of new antibiotics, I felt especially shitty. I got in bed a little early, which I almost never did—since I wouldn't fall asleep anyway.

As I lay down, I had a feeling similar to the time when I lost all control for hours in Utah. There was that warmth again, the pain leaving, seeing my dead best friend Spencer, my dead brother Nathan, and my dead grandfather Gilbert. Everything went white. The trio seemed happy to see me even though they were emotionless. It was as if they were there, but my eyes weren't producing them. I sensed, *It's your time, my guy,* like I was going on vacation. It was finally time for this to end. The warm fuzzy feeling enveloped me further, and I was happy to oblige.

I thought it was the end. I fell into a dreamless sleep.

I woke up confused. I had slept the whole night. No insomnia, no wide awake at 4:00 a.m. I felt better...I mean, I wasn't free from Lyme—but I wasn't in pure suffering either.

I was surprised I didn't die.

It was yet another experience I kept to myself.

* * *

I continued with all my treatments and protocols, and although my days were rough, I was still working. I wasn't as completely destroyed as I'd been before.

Could I be getting better?

Although I'd just seen dead people again and thought I died, I *was* slowly getting better. Like a stock graph going upward, there are still ups and downs, but the overall trend was slowly ascending. My brain fog was starting to lift. I was still sick, but something inside me was shifting.

One day in July of 2018, I drove east out of Phoenix. One part of the city, where I started, was covered in clouds and rain, while the other, distant part was cloudless and sunny. As I drove toward the clear and sunny part, I could see it slowly coming closer. I felt my mind gaining clarity while I got closer and closer to the light.

It felt like a spiritual experience. As I emerged from the overcast, my brain had the exact simulation of the outside world—like something straight out of a movie. Speeding along, I understood that I was going to beat Lyme. That I wasn't going to give up.

It was as if a part of my brain had been given back to me.

I could see the sunlit section nearing. I could see the clouds ending on the freeway and where the sun began. I was finally moving away from a dark daily experience of pain and suffering and moving toward relief instead. As I approached the sun, the music in my car enhanced my senses, all the while sparking a deep sense of change within me.

I had received an undeniable glimpse that I would feel better. And I *felt* better as I hit the sunlight. A feeling washed over me, reassuring me that one day I would get over this. Yes, I knew it might take a long time, but one day, *I would beat it.* My body and mind were moving toward relief and out of the foggy shit clouds of Lyme and coinfections as my car left behind the drear of the clouds and shot onto the sun-bathed highway.

To get better, I had to come to acceptance.

The denial of a chronic life-altering health condition was brutal. It took me years and years to fully accept it. Given what I've described here, you might wonder how I could not accept what was going on with me. The truth is, it is really hard to accept the reality that now, and maybe forever, your life sucks. Normally when we're sick with just a cold or flu we can look forward to getting better in a week or two. But to have the flu for years on end? I kept thinking I would get better. But I didn't. I really didn't want to accept that this was my life, period. That I couldn't travel. I couldn't exercise. That my life boiled down to surviving every day in anguish and despair, mostly alone.

It was very, very hard to accept that.

It was a very long time until those random "fuck everything" moments of anger and hatred dissipated, or at least were more spaced out. Then, as I finally accepted more and more of my situation, I considered what I could do with what I could control. I had to accept that if my life was a river, it was flowing in a direction I didn't want it to go. I was in a little boat and had been trying to row against the current. I had to accept that the current was going to take me where it wanted to. I had to accept my limitations, surrender to it, stop fighting it so much, and navigate the boat within that reality. And I should keep rowing.

When your success in recovery isn't exactly none,

But you're starting to accept the battle can't be 100 percent won.

You're trying to win the race, but this is something you can't outrun.

It's not failure to accept when a specific chapter of possibility is done.

Accepting it is better than so much pain of "I want to buy a handgun."

I gotta let go of the fact I used to be number one.

I don't have to be that person anymore to be someone.

A recreation of myself thinking of the long run.

Maybe less indoors and stress and more midnight sun.

Instead of visions of overworking to death, visions of future grandsons.

Maybe this is when I'll look back and see that my happiness truly began.

* * *

But Lyme wasn't done with me yet. A few months went by, and I was still living the roller coaster—some days way worse than others. I just couldn't take it anymore, and I broke again (are you noticing a pattern?).

I busted out some marijuana mints I got a long time ago. The mints were supposedly Sativa, which I don't like since it only increases the confusion and agony inside my brain, compared to indica, which provided more body relief. High-CBD, low-THC indica was the sweet spot. These mints? Super high Sativa. Whoops.

That night, I took not one but two of these mints. I didn't think they would be that strong since I'd had them for so long. Then I invited my friend Bryan out to watch a movie. A little bit into the movie, I knew what was coming. If I was getting that high that fast, I was in for a rough ride. *Here we go.*

I got so high my vision blurred. It felt like I was cross-eyed. I couldn't see the movie clearly, and I don't even remember what movie it was. I was high beyond reason.

After we left I got in my car so high that a kite could've looked up and still not seen me. I wouldn't have been able to compre-hend what a kite was anyway. I sat in the empty parking lot, rolled down my window, and recorded a video. It was 11:26 p.m. on a Sunday night, and I was freestyling about Lyme life into the camera.

I posted the video to Facebook and, like other posts, forgot that I did. The next day I woke up with a bunch of notifications. The video was over twelve minutes long; it had been shared sixty-two times, had 154 comments, and almost five thousand views. Oh shit. I guess people like the truth.

The video is here:

The comments, shares, and personal messages from that post let me know how many people out there need a voice. We all need one, but not everyone can straight up say how nightmarish their world is. Writing this book is risky. But someone has to do it.

* * *

I was still having a hard time maintaining a relationship. I might go on dates, but my health and the need to focus so much on myself kept getting in the way of sustaining anything. Then I met Brenda.

Brenda and I met through some weird dating app called Coffee Meets Bagel. I think I had half of all the dating apps in existence downloaded on my phone. We met at a random video game bar that I chose and had never been to. I learned that no matter how tired I was and how much I wished that dating could offer me a break from the fatigue and energy exertion of my entire existence, I still had to force the effort.

Brenda was Colombian, and although I told her it was just going to be a date and would lead to nothing else, we went back to my house.

After that, she kept hitting me up. I liked our connection. But what was interesting was her curiosity about my condition. It doesn't take long for someone to figure out that something is different with the person they are dating when there is a Rife machine emitting frequencies in the bed and an oxygen tank attached to an ozone machine with syringes in the living room corner; the kitchen cabinets are slammed with supplements; the bathtub has a million different detox items; and there is no kitchen table. Instead, there is just a giant four-person infrared sauna.

The more Brenda got to know me, the more she wanted to be around me. I was used to people being weirded out since I was still messed up. But I talked about Lyme confidently and freely with her. It felt like I was saying, "I have this thing that will drastically alter this relationship and make it so I can't do lots of things that you will want to do. By being with me, you will have to sacrifice us being able to do those things together."

That didn't seem to matter to her.

Brenda would grocery shop for me, cook me food, help me clean, cuddle with me, be there at night, go on my daily walks with me, and help me with my loneliness.

I am forever grateful for her.

Then her possessions accumulated in my apartment, and I got scared that she was trying to move in. So I made her remove all her stuff. This cycle repeated over and over—her trying to bring more stuff over and my telling her to take it back home. As you can tell, I have commitment issues.

Brenda was a lifesaver. Her heart was different from other people's. But we were not meant to be together. Although she cared about me deeply, and for a while our relationship was important to both of us, we were not able to create the kind of connection that a long-term relationship needs. We went our separate ways, but I will never forget her kindness.

CHAPTER
15

"I'm not faking being sick, I'm faking being well."

—UNKNOWN

BY THE LATE SUMMER OF 2018, I HAD CHANGED DOCTORS again. Dr. Mortell had been too aggressive with the testosterone prescription and had put me on a dangerous dose of Coartem. Other people told me they'd had bad experiences with him. I was losing trust.

I found a new MD, Dr. Traeger, who got me on a new cocktail of clarithromycin and Bactrim. I felt a bit better and more functional as the days went on. I'd been on antibiotics for a really long time, and if I hadn't taken a ton of probiotics and prebiotics and eaten the right foods, I'm sure my stomach would have been ruined.

In the meantime, I also was losing trust in how the company where I worked in Phoenix was being run. I mentioned to a coworker that I was thinking about starting my own solar sales firm, and we agreed to meet for dinner to discuss it. I chose an Ethiopian spot called Café Lalibela on University Drive in Tempe. As dinner time approached, I had a hard time getting up and walking around and had a weird malaise all over. I lived only ten minutes away from the restaurant, but I didn't know if I was going to be able to make it.

To give myself the boost I needed, I opened my fridge and drank a whole bottle of turmeric-flavored Wild Tonic Kombucha alcohol. It didn't take away all the pain and fatigue, so I took a couple of hits from a marijuana joint. For myself, one hit on a joint messes me up. I took two big hits and the pain began subsiding, but now I felt a bit detached from reality.

By the time I arrived at the restaurant I was pretty gone. As my head swam, I remembered how most of the time people can't tell how you are feeling on the inside. So I repeated to myself, *Nobody will notice that I am high and sick.*

We made the decision to start a solar sales company. I came up with the name Direct Solar, and we established on September 26, 2018. Soon we met with the installer, a company whose competing quotes I kept seeing while I was out selling. We met up with the business relations person, Jerry, and talked about doing business together. My new business partner told Jerry that I was one of the best salespeople he knew and that I would only get better as my health improved. Jerry then asked, "What's going on with your health?"

"I have Lyme."

"My friend had Lyme!" he said.

"How is he doing now?"

"He felt horrible all the time, that he was a burden on his wife and family, so one night he got in his hot tub and shot himself."

He told me this as if he were talking about the weather. I was shocked, but I felt bad for the guy. I often wanted to do the same thing. Afterward, my business partner was pissed off about it, but I told him it didn't bother me and that Jerry was just trying to relate.

It was super exciting to be selling deals for my own company and making a lot more money on top of it. The only thing that was weird was how my business partner and I had agreed to split the profits of the first five sales—they were to be invested back into the company. But I was the only one selling deals. My partner wasn't. That was my first red flag.

When a couple more salespeople joined us in Arizona to start training, I quickly realized my partner wasn't doing anything on the back end, either. My friend Matt called me to see how I was, I told him I'd started Direct Solar, and he said he wanted to join us. He showed up in a few days and became the VP of sales in Las Vegas.

I became very, very busy because I was helping train and support the Las Vegas team from Phoenix, running the show in Arizona from my apartment, and still occasionally selling my own deal.

There were days I couldn't use the bathroom because there was no time due to all the phone calls. It was insane. Brenda totally took care of me. I would sit at home working all day long and executing all my health routines. At one point, she literally picked up a fork and directly fed me by putting it in my mouth as I pounded away at my keyboard. Even though my health took unpredictable turns, I could keep the worst of my symptoms at bay with Brenda taking care of me.

* * *

And then I developed a horrifying new symptom.

I had heard people describe vertigo, but as is the case with anything, you never really know what it's like until you live it. I hate nausea. Vertigo is extreme nausea plus spinning.

When it struck, I couldn't do anything. It was game over. I tried everything I could to get it to stop: lying on my side to reposition ear crystals, deep breathing exercises, and so on, but nothing helped. The room never spun an entire circle; it did this half-circle thing, back and forth.

Vertigo was hell.

One day, when I thought it had calmed down, I went out to meet with a potential customer my partner had given me. She was a tough cookie. I'd gathered all my data and prepped everything for the close.

As I sat at her kitchen table, I noticed I was sweating more than usual. That was one of the warning signs. I thought, *Oh boy, not now.*

I tried to keep it together and attempted to breathe deeply, but my face dripped sweat, and I only got dizzier.

"Have you ever had vertigo before?" I asked her.

"Yes," she said. The look on her face told me she was a bit worried.

"Well, I am about to have a full-on vertigo episode." She stared back in silence.

I couldn't function. I got up from her kitchen table and slumped on a chair in the corner.

"Do you need anything?" she asked.

"I'm going to throw up."

As she grabbed a little bucket, I slid down the chair to sit on the ground. It wasn't helping. I took the little bucket and started puking in it. I couldn't do anything but ride it out in some random stranger's house.

As I crouched on the floor, beaten by the waves of nausea and retching helplessly, I could hear her in the other room on the phone with a friend. She talked softly, but I still caught every word: "I have a solar guy here, and he is just sitting on the floor throwing up and dizzy... What do I do?"

I texted my business partner and asked him to pick me up. He and his daughter came to get me so that he could drive my Corolla and she could drive me back to their place in their car.

The entire drive I was sick and fighting mounting nausea. I tried to breathe through it, but that didn't do anything. Thirty minutes later I was still sick. I sat in his driveway and chewed on some mango he gave me, hoping the vertigo would pass.

At last, although I wasn't all the way recovered, I used all my strength to drive home. I collapsed onto the couch on my side and prayed for relief.

My mind was gripped by fear. *Holy shit. Am I developing a new symptom that is going to completely alter my life? Am I going to get these episodes while driving? If I get stressed or am in a house, will I now have to deal with this for the rest of my life?*

Luckily, the vertigo subsided after two weeks. I haven't had one episode since. I don't know where the vertigo came from, why it happened, and if it was stress-induced from running the business or what, but I am damn grateful that I haven't been struck by any more episodes. Just writing about it creeps me out. Vertigo puts you on your knees and controls you for a good two hours. I wouldn't wish that condition on anyone.

* * *

With my vertigo resolved, I refocused on taking care of my mental health. I asked around in the Facebook Lyme groups for a good therapist and got a recommendation for an EMDR therapist in Scottsdale. I started EMDR with Dr. Allman when I lived in San Diego, and it did me a lot of good. But when I moved back to Utah, I dropped it. I didn't make the effort to find a good practitioner there.

But I knew there was a lot in my head to process. Doing EMDR allowed me to step out of how I had compartmentalized and numbed everything out, so I would be forced to actually deal with my emotions. I felt a lot of sadness, fear, and anger. I was white-knuckling through every day, just compartmentalizing and trying to get through. EMDR allowed me to feel my feelings, to stop suppressing them. When I did that, I started to be able to deal with them. Until I did that work, I was dissociating from the pain and trauma I had experienced and was continuing to experience with Lyme. Sometimes I felt more "real" after doing EMDR, if that makes sense. Dissociating was the way my brain protected me and helped me get through, but it kept me in a traumatized place.

After an EMDR session, I'd feel more complete, more aware of my emotions. I had a clearer mind and could see things differently. It was always beneficial. If I hadn't undergone EMDR, I wouldn't have been able to run the business or the other aspects of my life.

I've never fully understood why people wouldn't want to do therapy. Why wouldn't you want someone to help you mentally and emotionally if those are major drivers of our entire lives?

* * *

As the Vegas office improved, I realized Arizona wasn't doing that well and that my partner wasn't doing anything. There wasn't a real need for him. I like to be loyal to people and not abandon them, but I got the sense that he was chilling at the pool all day while I worked my ass off. I started to feel frustrated, manipulated, and screwed over.

I work in and on relationships all the time. Being good at reading people is essential to being a good salesperson. Yet, maybe due to Lyme brain fog, I found myself in partnership with someone who really was not good for me. It seemed to me that he wanted me to do all the work while he sat back. Looking back, I knew I should have seen that something was off. I should have been a better judge of character, but being sick blunted my ability to do that.

I knew I had to change the situation.

I met up with him at a Starbucks just before Thanksgiving, just two months after we started Direct Solar, and let him know I didn't think he was a good fit. Things weren't working between us. I said I planned to buy him out and keep the Direct Solar name.

He did not take it well. I was prepared for that, but for the next two weeks, as we worked to disentangle our business, he issued subtle threats around burning my apartment down and murdering me. In the end, I paid him $50,000 and the business was mine. I was not surprised that right after I bought him out he registered "Direct Solar and Batteries" and launched his own company.

Paying him off meant I wouldn't make any money for a while. In the first year of operations, I actually reported negative income. I worked my ass off for free for months.

I traveled from Phoenix to Las Vegas for the company holiday party at the end of 2018. Most of the people working in that office had not met me in person, so I knew I had to show up strong. I knew they all were going to be watching and judging me.

I was nervous. Travel is hard on my body, and I had to make a good impression. I dressed well and joined the Christmas party. Everyone was watching my every move, judging what I said and how I said it. Every part of me was in the spotlight, and despite not feeling good, I thugged it out and came off as charismatic and put-together. People couldn't tell what was going on inside. I hid how bad I felt and pretended to be normal even though I was far from it.

I focused more and more on the Las Vegas market and began driving over regularly. (I finally moved there full time in the fall of 2019.) In the beginning, I could only stay a maximum of three days at a time. Each time I visited, I tested myself to see how long I could stay without collapsing and having to go home. It was a way of measuring to see if I was getting better.

Once, I just couldn't generate the strength to lead a sales meeting. But I couldn't let anyone see me that sick. I told my VP I had to go home to Arizona immediately. Nobody knew I had Lyme, and I didn't tell anyone either. I just kept thugging it out, pretending everything was normal, convinced I had gotten away with my ruse. As I drove home to Arizona, I was a bit defeated by my limitations, but I knew the truth was I had Lyme, and I couldn't control it.

CHAPTER
16

"I don't think anyone really understands how tiring it is to act okay and always be 'strong' when in reality you're close to the edge."

—UNKNOWN

IN FEBRUARY 2019, DR. TRAEGER TOLD ME IT WAS TIME to come off antibiotics. I wasn't sure that was a good idea since I was trying to run my business and the clarithromycin and Bactrim combo seemed to be helping me. She said I would eventually need to come off antibiotics, and this would be a good test.

Under my doctor's advice, I went off the antibiotics and within days was absolutely DESTROYED. *Oh my god, I just want to die again.*

All my Lyme symptoms rushed back to the surface.

I was desperate once more.

But I had something else to try.

Shortly before I ditched my meds, members in the old Utah Lyme support group had told me about a hyperthermia clinic in Bountiful, Utah. Feeling like hell now, I called the clinic.

Hyperthermia is supposed to kill pathogens with heat. Supposedly, Lyme in a petri dish stops moving at a specific temperature, sheds its exoskeleton when the temperature gets a little bit warmer, and starts to die at around 103.5 degrees. It was a competition to see how much internal heat I could tolerate and how much the Lyme could tolerate.

The goal is to get really hot but not go past 107 degrees, which can cause brain damage.

The clinic also treated cancer patients. Pathogens and cancer hate heat and oxygen, so they flooded cancer patients with a massive induced fever and lots of oxygen. People from the Lyme support group who had already undergone the treatment told me it was one of the hardest things they had ever done in their lives. I heard what they said but didn't believe it. I had done a lot of hard things.

The clinic told me they didn't have any openings for a while. What they didn't know was that I intended to come in that week. I was going to tour their place to determine if I was going to do their treatment or not. When they repeated that they didn't think they could fit me in, I stated firmly, "You don't understand. I am flying in on Thursday. I can see your place on Friday to decide if I am going to enroll in your treatment. What time do you have on Friday to see me?"

The person could hear in the tone of my voice that I wasn't messing around. She set the appointment. When it is life or death, it is life or death. When someone absolutely NEEDS to make something happen, it will happen, no matter what. The two-week treatment was going to cost $5,000, but I didn't care. When you are that sick, you will do whatever you have to.

When I visited, the clinic staff told me they had a success rate of 90 percent, which probably wasn't true, but their confidence was still reassuring. I booked my first consultation for the next week.

I told Matt, my VP, what I was doing and that I couldn't answer the phone until 2:00–3:00 p.m. most days since I would be in treatment. Nobody else in the company knew what I was doing.

On the day I needed to make that long drive to Utah, I woke up completely annihilated. I knew what was ahead of me and every fiber and ounce of my soul thought I couldn't make that drive from Phoenix, Arizona, to Salt Lake City, Utah. But I had to. I used all my willpower to get out of bed.

To give me the strength to get to Utah, I looked at my Carlos fingerprint dog tag, took a quarter of a marijuana gummy, and started my drive. Driving long distances was incredibly taxing; taking a marijuana gummy eased the stress. I never took a whole gummy—just enough to take the edge off the Lyme.

I began the drive as the marijuana kicked in, so tired I leaned over my steering wheel, barely able to focus. As I powered through, I felt like I had endured ten hours of drive time within the first thirty minutes. I was going to suffer the whole way. As I drove, I bawled my eyes out for an hour; I was in so much pain and all alone, making the trek by myself. I didn't know how I was going to make it, but I was.

*　*　*

I stayed in Utah with my father and his wife, Colleen. She dropped me off at the clinic on the first day.

I drank a special smoothie, then got on a bike to go hard for one minute, medium intensity for two minutes, switching back and forth for a total of ten minutes. I hadn't been able to exercise in a long time, so this was incredibly taxing on my body. The smoothie they gave me had niacin and B vitamins in it, which made me feel weird. Not to mention the oxygen I was hooked up to had me looking like a total Lyme patient. After all that, I went downstairs to a scary-looking chamber with a table that had tubes all over it and a bunch of medical equipment surrounding it.

Several nurses were waiting for me. There was a TV on the ceiling and a skintight, zip-up suit on a hanger. I put it on and was strapped down to the table.

I felt like I was in a movie. I had no idea what to expect. The person in charge of monitoring my vitals turned on a random television show. As they started the treatment, hot water flowed into the suit. It wasn't so hot that I felt that it was going to hurt me, but it was hot enough that I knew I was going to feel it. At first it even felt good.

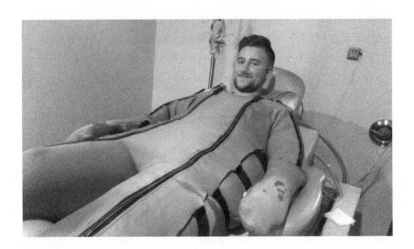

After about five minutes, I thought I was golden. But then... *Damn,* that's *some hot water.* My whole body was engulfed. I was trapped in the suit, with oxygen going in my nose and only a TV for distraction. When I got to the ten-minute mark everything went fuzzy. I started to lose control as I pushed my paranoid thoughts to the side and tried to focus on the show. But shit...*I don't understand what's going on with the TV.*

Everything blurred together. *I am a prisoner in this suit.* I was delirious. I fought to find mental strength, thinking about what I was going through. It was like when you run a marathon and hit the wall. Previously, when I was suffering, every minute felt like an hour. In the suit, every minute felt like two hours. Now I understood why other patients had told me that doing this treatment was one of the hardest tasks they had ever undertaken in their entire lives.

I tried surrendering to it, telling myself it would be only a little bit longer, but I still had a long way to go. As I neared the mid-point of the treatment, I shook and twitched, almost like I was seizing. My head rolled side to side, side to side, side to side.

One nurse remarked, "I can't understand how the treatment can be so hard."

"Well," I managed to say in between thrashing, "have you ever done it?"

She hadn't.

I was dazed after it was over. I needed a long time to sit up and get off the table. Next, they sent me into a massive electromagnetic machine to vibrate my body, knock more of the bad pathogens out, and kill it off. Finally, I had to sit in a chair for an IV, do a BrainTap meditation to calm down (which involved wearing headphones with a visor over my eyes that played a guided meditation while flashing lights hit my closed eyelids), then stand on a vibration plate.

The whole process bottomed me out. But I did feel better. I had less pain throughout my body.

The thing was, I had to come back and do it again. And again. And again, for two weeks.

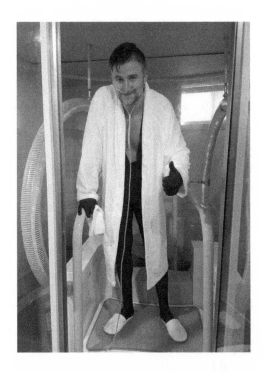

Sometimes the nurses talked about the procedure as if I wasn't there. Sometimes, they would get nervous or freak out about a reading on my vitals. Eventually, I told them it wasn't professional for them to lose their cool. I needed everything in my power to make it through this damn treatment—including their confident attitudes.

One day, when I was in the IV room, I grabbed the arm of one of the newer nurses I liked. I told her I had to have her there with me during all my treatments and to please put in that request with her superiors. I stared deeply into her eyes. She was the only one I trusted—the one who I felt comfortable having next to me. I could tell that the human part of her was still intact. It hadn't been numbed out yet by watching people go through the treatments every day.

In the third session, I had to stop early. I felt like a failure, thinking I was supposed to be able to tough it out, but I couldn't. That day was a waste to me.

By the fifth day—the last day of that first week—it was so hard I got in my car afterward and cried. I didn't know how I was going to continue. Colleen told me she would come in to support me. I had no idea how I was going to finish the treatment, but I knew I had to. If it would fix my Lyme, it had to be done.

To hack the pain, I started to take a little marijuana gummy before each session even though the clinic told me not to. I didn't know how else to take the edge off. Once, I took a little bit more, and all the THC did was enhance how hardcore the treatment was. I learned not to do that.

Hyperthermia treatment lasts about forty-five to fifty minutes, but it was a mental endurance test each and every time. The hottest my internal temperature ever got to was 105 degrees.

Colleen had ice-cold hands. By simply placing her hands on my forehead she gave me instant relief.

Once, my father came to watch, but it was too much for him. I think it gave him flashbacks to watching Nathan dying from cancer. I felt like I had to support him while he watched me in the treatment. Ultimately, having him there made it harder for me. I preferred the cold hands of Colleen.

Toward the end of the second week, the staff showed me how to replicate the hyperthermia treatment in a hot tub so I could continue on my own. After we did the hot tub session I felt so good I did pushups and swam laps in the pool. I wanted to feel like that all the time and was optimistic yet again that the treatment would help me in the long run. I felt real relief from the despair that had plagued me for so long.

* * *

Successfully completing that hyperthermia treatment made me feel like I'd gone through a mini Navy SEAL mental fortitude boot camp. After I finished the treatment in Utah, knowing I had knocked the number of spirochetes in my blood down, I headed to Tijuana, Mexico, to get a stem cell injection. This time, the doctors said my infection rates were low enough for the stem cells to work.

Stem cells seemed to help me for about three weeks after each treatment. I'd have a little more energy, a little less inflammation. Right after I got the injection, I usually had a really good night's sleep. The way stem cells work, they could repair tissues that had been damaged by inflammation and the infection. That was good—I needed to keep my symptoms under control so I could keep building my business—but stem cells didn't really get me better, since they didn't do anything to actually get rid of the Lyme. The stem cells repair the damage that the Lyme has caused. That's why the hyperthermia, which focused on killing off spirochetes, made sense to me, and doing stem cells after the Lyme count was reduced would help increase the stem cells' effectiveness.

When I got home, I began doing hyperthermia treatments on my own. The goal is to get my body temperature over 102 degrees, preferably over 102.5 degrees, and keep it there for twenty minutes.

It was almost harder doing it at home than it was at the clinic. Afterward, I would jump on a trampoline for ten minutes to stimulate my lymphatic system. I bought oxygen canisters to breathe in pure oxygen at the peak of the session and after the session to try to kill the Lyme.

There was a learning curve as I figured out how to do the hyperthermia myself. For one, bathtubs are far superior to hot tubs. Once I had the bath so hot that I burned my feet, but I pushed through it. After that, I ordered a meat thermometer to use in the bathwater, so I could keep the water at 115 degrees and prevent any future burns.

By this time, I was doing the treatment five times a week at my house and finding the process just as hard as doing it at the clinic. You are supposed to have someone watching you, but I rarely did.

CHAPTER
17

"The purpose of life is not to be happy. It is to be useful, to be honorable, to be compassionate, to have it make some difference that you have lived and lived well."

—RALPH WALDO EMERSON

AFTER THAT HYPERTHERMIA TREATMENT IN UTAH, I WAS off antibiotics for about eight months, which was amazing. I had been on antibiotics for eighteen months straight, since I moved to Utah in 2017, which wasn't good. They aren't something you should take long-term because they are like a flamethrower to your gut flora. I had a lot of negative reactions to them, lots of stomach problems, ringing in the ears, and so on. But whenever I tried to get off them I'd just be flattened by the disease. I wouldn't even be able to get out of bed. Almost completely collapsing is worse than being on antibiotics. I understand now that they play a critical role in recovery for a lot of people with Lyme and coinfections. No one person is the same or has the same journey of stuff that works for them individually.

I was still having lots of ups and downs, but it was a miracle to not be dependent on antibiotics anymore. My gut could finally start to heal itself. In the fall of 2019, I did have to get back on antibiotics for a while to knock the disease back again, but the hyperthermia I kept doing at home definitely was working.

Although I was healing, anytime I got excited and went a bit too hard, I was punished instantly. It's a weird feeling having that rev limiter on. I could hardly eat anything and couldn't lift weights or exercise at all. When I looked in the mirror, I saw how my muscles had shrunk away, but I couldn't do anything about it. I couldn't go at my goals as hard as I wanted to, so I had to mentally pivot and do what I *could* do, knowing that others might judge, but doing it anyway.

* * *

During the summer of 2019, the business became increasingly stressful. We were losing reps because my VP—my old friend Matt—was still handling a lot of the functions of the business in Vegas and was doing things like handwriting checks to our salespeople with no real accuracy. They didn't know if they were being paid on time and/or correctly. That meant I had to spend more and more time in Vegas. I kept telling Matt what needed to change but he wouldn't listen, so I had to put a stop to it and take over the payroll.

One of the most humbling experiences in my life was losing my mental capacities. At this point in the timeline, I was still messed up and not all there, but being at 30 percent was better than being at 10 percent. At 30 percent, I could read a bit and make more accurate decisions. I knew I was going to have to manage the stress or the Lyme would come roaring back. I needed these skills because all at once, I was dealing with multiple business angles, legal issues, hiring, sales management, others trying to attack my business, building an online web presence, running sales meetings and trainings, and so on. The mental stimulation of having to solve complex issues was nice. It was difficult and strenuous, but man, so much better than not being able to work.

A sales meeting is public speaking. As the founder of Direct Solar, I had to get up and give motivational speeches to the sales team several times a week while I felt like shit and wanted to die. I had all this stuff going on with my body and my brain that I believed I had to hide. A leader is always on stage. Everything they do constantly trickles down to everyone else. I had to appear strong and motivated, even when I felt weak and unmotivated. If I was weak and unmotivated, then they would be weak and unmotivated.

Our whole company was about sales, and all the salespeople depended on me to lead them. I believed I couldn't let anyone see me as sick or weak. If they saw the owner ill, they would lose faith and confidence. Sometimes I had to inject Toradol, which is like very strong aspirin, before I ran a sales meeting. I couldn't take it very often because that would risk organ damage. But I knew I had to be on my game.

Sales meetings are extra intense because the audience is all salespeople, and they watch every move. They judge me. Based on how I run a meeting, they are going to believe in me and the company and go out and sell hard, or they are going to doubt me and the company, and not sell. Maybe look for something else. If they don't believe what I'm saying, they're not going to work here.

Consequently, I put myself under enormous pressure to perform. I felt all the success of the company rested on my shoulders. If I didn't perform and inspire, nobody would do their job, and the company would fail. I had to get up and essentially save the company every single sales meeting, even on days when I barely could get out of bed and was actively thinking about blowing my brains out. Sometimes in the beginning I would be the only one posting to the group chat and signing deals. I had to do it for a week straight by myself for others to jump on. I had not just the weight of the company but the weight of Lyme all bearing down on me simultaneously. Each one by themselves is hard enough; I had to carry both.

The business is really simple. We go door-to-door to sell people residential solar power systems. Once we sell a system, we contract with a solar installation company to fulfill the engineering, permits, and work. All we do is the sales part.

I was doing the job of four people and had to go to Tijuana for stem cells every three months just to give myself a little boost that lasted only three to four weeks. Everything I was doing came down to pure survival mode, but Lyme and the rest of my life taught me how to survive. There were no safety nets, and nobody was there to save the day except my therapist, who heard my crazy stories, and Taylor and TJ to pick up the rest of the mental slack.

I got some support from great friends like Jonny, Jeff, Trey, Cody, Yajaira, Gavin, Justin, and a few others, but I kept 95 percent of my struggles to myself.

* * *

I knew I was doing better when I realized I hadn't had a suicidal thought in a couple of months. It might seem as if I talk about suicidal thoughts nonchalantly, and suicide has been a major reoccurring theme in this book, but Lyme made them normal. The suicidal thoughts became background noise I lived with and got used to. They were a side effect of my brain not working right. It was only when they got stronger that I knew I had to do something to make the urge quieter.

When the business in Vegas devolved into a bad situation with Matt over the summer of 2019, I decided I had to move there to save it, so I relocated to Summerlin, Nevada. Everything I owned fit in my car. I told one of the sales reps that wanted to move out of Matt's house, "Find a house in Las Vegas for us to rent, this week, no matter what. I don't care what it is. Just find it." Then we moved in, and I went to work. All I did when I lived there was wake up, attend to business and sales all day, then do it again. There was no "off" or "me" time at all. I lived on raw business day in and day out.

This was murder on my body. Randomly, Lyme knocked me down and I felt like shit. When that happened, I would hide so other people wouldn't know how sick I was. I would work from my bed and still get everything done, but I didn't want them to see the state I was in. I could fully wish for death in that moment and see a phone call coming in, turn on the enthusiasm for five minutes, then go back to my misery, so they wouldn't know. But it gets really hard to keep that to yourself when you are living with people.

The business was so demanding, it made me sick. I realized I was having another problem with Matt—he was so stressful to work with that I would get Lyme flare-ups.. I tried to fix this by seeing my EMDR therapist every time I went to Arizona. I'd clear up some emotions, let out all the pressure and stress, have someone hear out all the actual things that were going on in my world, then get back after it.

It came to a head when I concluded I had to fire Matt. We met in September 2019. It took an hour to have this difficult conversation with him. When I said, "We have to part ways. This isn't working anymore," a couple of tears leaked out of my eyes.

That was a hard conversation. I viewed Matt as a good friend.

I knew it was the right decision, and it had to be done if I was going to save the business and myself. I didn't know if I would still have a team, though, after he left, since he had relationships with them. I had to go run a sales meeting a few days later. I was about to find out.

When I walked in, almost every single person was there, on time and ready to listen. I was shocked and humbled. These people trusted me. I felt a deep sense of purpose. They reaffirmed that if I stuck to solid principles, to treating people right and caring for them, and having the mindset that I worked for them and not them for me, I could succeed in the long run. My body still had quite a way to go to catch up from all the stress of breaking my business relationship with Matt, but the possibility was real that the business could get better and some of the stress might lessen.

I was getting better at the sales meetings, but they were still super hard, especially when I woke up after the nightly Lyme train ran my ass over. Most people couldn't tell when I felt like I was going to pass out during a meeting. During one meeting, as I was looking out in the crowd and teaching sales, I thought to myself, *Holy shit. I might pass out right now. Hopefully, I don't.* Later, when I became more open with people at work about my health in late 2019, several of them said they suspected something was really wrong—they thought I had cancer, and the hyperthermia treatment I did was to treat it.

The anxiety caused by Lyme and public speaking combined with feeling sick while having to run an hour-and-a-half *engaging* and *motivating* sales meeting is a whole other beast. To get through hard stuff like this in the business, I recommitted to my principles.

My principles helped me get out of my head by focusing on others. They were, and are, these:

- It's not about me, it's about them.

- Figure out how to provide the most value.

- Figure out how to help others.

I recommitted to the right focus. That's how I made it work. With Lyme, you have to go to the deepest core of your being to make it work sometimes.

Part of my healing journey has been recognizing that if I focus on other people, rather than myself, I feel better. One of the reasons building my business was so important was because I want to use it to help people, especially the people who work for me. I have since broadened that understanding out to my desire to help people in the Lyme community. I know what despair and loneliness feel like. I empathize with that. I began to work toward the idea of using my achievements and my talents to be the person who could be there, even metaphorically, for another Lyme sufferer. This became one of the carrots I placed in front of myself during dark times. I was going to get through this so I could help other people get through it too.

I took more people under my wing to help them succeed in the game of sales, and I learned something important about myself. I was having a blast! Getting your own sale is fun. Helping change someone's life so they increase their sales is more exciting than closing your own deals. If I took my focus off myself and concentrated on how I could deliver the most value to our salespeople and help them succeed, I could forget about my suffering, pain, and pure shitty situation.

I became hooked on helping people and boosting them up. I wanted to train everyone and made myself available twenty-four seven. Not only was I running the office, but I was out knocking doors and racking up sales; I was saving deals when it was needed. I still had to pace myself, and be careful, but damn it felt good to do so much—when I hadn't been able to keep up before.

Every day, I poured my heart and soul into helping everyone around me so I could forget about myself. My coping mechanism was helping my sales reps succeed. That was the best escape from my pain.

There's nothing like the joy of transforming your team's lives so they can get out of debt, send money to their families, and improve their lives. There's nothing like hearing them tell you how much their job means to them. The impact feels amazing.

I didn't just make it my goal to give all I could to the current business; I set myself up so I could give on higher levels than I ever had. What I was doing was a lot deeper than just "working." Selling solar saved my life.

* * *

Things get weird as you start to improve your life. As I began to heal, some old friends started treating me differently.

My friend Lacy, who had helped me when I nearly killed myself in my garage, had always believed that Lyme was a lifelong thing, and I couldn't fix it. When she saw me getting better, that messed with her reality. She ghosted me—even though I often had been there for her. When I asked her why she did, she said she "had her reasons." When I asked her what those were, she told me, "I can't believe you'd ask me that during a pandemic," and then blocked me on everything.

I was giving and giving and giving and giving, and that was so rewarding. But sometimes I would ask myself, *When is it my turn?* Sometimes I desperately wanted to be around people who didn't need something from me, so I could relax. Being selfless and helping people had become my mission. Still, you have to remember to take care of yourself. Who was going to be there for me the way I was there for them?

I developed a more truthful "reality" versus a "positive thinking" way of seeing my healing with Lyme and the world at large. I was still spending a lot of time each week on my health. I worked all day every day and still spent probably thirty hours a week on health-related stuff. There was just moving forward; there was no such thing as downtime.

Whatever I was doing was slowly working. I was getting a little bit sharper each day. Today, I can't even fully comprehend the level of suffering I felt in San Diego. When I had bad days in late 2019, I reminded myself, *My bad days are still better than my good days back then.*

One of the biggest takeaways I learned through becoming one of the top door-to-door salesmen in the country for SolarCity and starting to heal from Lyme is that the hardcore positive thinking trend is dangerous. I've closely watched successful people get there through a will to win and pure hustle. I can't stress enough that that is a dangerous mindset to have with Lyme.

I'll just say it: going to a Tony Robbins event won't cure your Lyme.

You can't simply think that your body is already healthy and that you'll wake up healthy tomorrow and boom! You're better.

Putting up a healthy version of you on a vision board won't fix you, either, although it is a good thing to have.

Whenever I question these things out loud, people conclude that I'm against positive thinking, when I'm not. I went to EMDR therapy twice a week for months to make sure negative emotional states weren't lowering my immune system. I had a vision board on my wall in San Diego, although most of it was covered in pictures of dogs and puppies. I do believe in positive thinking, but on its own, it's not enough.

The real gems in self-help are found by wading through all the bullshit. Sales reps who obsessively studied similar theories to the Law of Attraction never sold much solar. The high sellers had a strong mindset to win combined with a killer work ethic. When I got sick, the people obsessed with self-help were the first ones to abandon me.

We don't need "positive thinking." We need "accurate thinking." I had conversations with certain close friends in which I said things that would make a positive thinker gasp, such as, "My life is horrifically shitty right now," and "I have no idea how I have survived this long." I left relieved after those talks and felt I could develop an actual game plan to change what I was doing in my life so I would get better.

It's weird that saying "My life sucks" helped improve my life more than trying to fake the opposite. Maybe that's all you need sometimes—to just take the mask off and say, "Screw it, I'm going to be honest right now about my life and stop suppressing my terrible thoughts."

It's not accurate to think that a disease is incurable. It's also not accurate to think we can't colonize Mars. Both things can *seem* almost impossible, but they aren't. Of course, you don't want to plan on haphazardly putting together a rocket ship and making it to Mars using only "positive thinking." If this is what you want to do, you better be prepared for some rough conditions. Even Elon Musk said that he thought his company Tesla would fail based on the statistics, but he did it anyway.

Even if you could accomplish feats like that, it's not accurate to think you can cure your cancer overnight or fly on a paper plane with Elon Musk through the galaxy and make it to the red planet. You can't do that. You can't buy a plant and only chant affirmations at it to keep it alive. You have to actually water the plant.

CHAPTER
18

"You've got to make tough decisions, sometimes unpopular decisions... Whatever it is, if it's the right move at the right time, you've got to be also willing to make mistakes."

—SEAN MCDERMOTT

I JOINED A LAS VEGAS SUPPORT GROUP AFTER SOMEONE referred me to SOT (Supportive Oligonucleotide Therapy). This infusion therapy is designed to prevent the Lyme bacteria from replicating by creating a molecule that blocks an important function of the bacteria's DNA. One of the members of the group, AJ, told me he had good success with the therapy. Although it takes a long time to feel the benefits of it, he said he felt great most days. I could tell he was used to people being skeptical.

I wasn't. Although I had learned that the roller coaster of optimism was usually followed by the pain of disappointment and failure, I still had hope. People with Lyme get jaded. When you hear of someone who got better, you don't want to believe it because you don't want to be let down again. AJ quickly saw how open I was to the idea. I joined SOT Facebook groups and started researching it and found a number of success stories.

One old acquaintance I hadn't talked to in a long time randomly hit me up saying that her friend had done SOT, and it had made a huge difference for her. The cost was $5,000 plus lab work and other stuff. After I heard that, doing SOT was an easy decision. I was determined to try it.

I saw this opportunity as being no different than if I went down to a casino on the Vegas strip, and someone said, "If you put $5,000 on this roulette table, you have a 10 percent chance of healing your Lyme." I would make that bet every...single...time. That's a no-brainer. I'd already spent a lot more than that trying to get better.

I have long been ready to pay someone a million dollars and go into debt to cure my Lyme. People think doing a coffee enema or sleeping with lights from a Rife bulb in my bed is weird? Who cares? If that stuff made a measurable mark in my progress, I would do it every damn day. Paying for treatment was easy.

I contacted the clinic in late 2019 and let them know I wanted to set up a time to talk to the doctor. I had to complete lab work before I could get the treatment in Atlanta. The wait to get the lab work took four agonizing months.

Those four months felt like forever. I was going through different antibiotics, dealing with different coinfections, and getting torn up. Was the problem now Bartonella? Was it Babesia? Was it my high strep levels? The doctor did extensive testing. He found pathogens I had never seen or heard of before. I went on Nystatin for a long time and cut out fermented foods and kombucha to help bring my yeast to the lowest possible levels in my gut. I looked at my hormonal levels in different ways.

Running meetings was still hard; I still had brain fog, pain, fatigue, and depression, and life was still incredibly hard. It just wasn't *as hard* as it was before. I went from pure hell to mere hell. Now, even though I was still in hell, I could function. I knew I was slowly getting better.

At last, in March of 2020, I went to see Dr. Hartzmann, the physician in Georgia who would conduct the Supportive Oligonucleotide Therapy. As I stepped off the plane, I was excited. This was my chance to take something to help myself. As I was hopeful, I also knew to stay level-headed. I'd had a lot of roller coaster rides.

I had my Google drive folder labeled "Health History"ready with all my labwork, organized by date taken and the description. All I have to do is share that link with a doctor, and they instantly have an easily searchable database comprising a timeline of all my tests. I also keep a history of all my symptoms and have recorded how much sleep I got with key changes in medications and supplements. This makes it easy for my doctors to find trends.

I also brought a folder full of printed out test results just in case the doctor preferred hard copies versus digital copies. I had pictures loaded up on my phone from skin marks I had experienced to show him. I had questions and specific talking points written down to cover in my notes, and directions I thought might work best. I went in thinking about him and what he needed from me to work efficiently.

On some tests, I'd tabbed the page that I knew he would want to see so he could quickly get there. I had the tests I knew he wanted up front and the others in the back just in case. A doctor is only with you for an hour each month. You are with yourself for 720 hours per month. It's impossible for them to know what's going on unless you work with them, offer suggestions, keep records, do what they tell you to do, and work as partners toward getting you better.

After talking for an hour, he told me that when I got better, I might as well become a Lyme doctor since I'd gone so in-depth with everything he needed to know, and I was already so far ahead. He also said he was almost "giddy" to get me better since I came in prepared the way I did. Having an enthusiastic doctor who wants to help you will do a lot more for you than a doctor neutral to your results.

Dr. Hartzmann gave me a lot of confidence in the procedure. Supposedly Lyme has an eighty- to ninety-day reproduction cycle. Since the SOT works through the use of a single nucleotide attaching to the pathogen and stopping it from replicating, it would take a while to reduce the Lyme pathogen load.

The SOT injection was simple, just a little tube of material injected into my saline bag on an IV. It came in a small tube that I still carry in my pocket today.

AJ, who had first recommended SOT, told me I wouldn't truly know if it worked for a while, so I was prepared for the long haul. Dr. Hartzmann told me to stay on my current antibiotic for four to six weeks and then stop. That scared the shit out of me. I had bad experiences going off antibiotics in the past. If I went off and got wrecked, Direct Solar could tank. It was a risky move. It felt too early. But the doctor assured me I would be OK. I saw it as a test to see if the treatment was real or not.

After about forty-five days I went off the antibiotic. The night before, I went to sleep knowing the next day I would be going off. Sometimes you have to surrender to whatever may happen and brace yourself. I imagined surrendering was like someone who has to cross a guarded trail in a war. They know they have to stay calm; they know they could get shot, but they also might not. So you walk across, hoping you don't get wiped out. You just look forward and do what you have to do.

I went off the antibiotic and...I didn't get wrecked! This was huge. I was expecting a complete shutdown and for all the Lyme that was hiding in me to come out with a vengeance, but it didn't.

This was about the same time the coronavirus pandemic started, in early 2020. Everything was going crazy. Businesses everywhere were shutting down. I had to stay strong for my team. I wasn't sure what was going to happen, but I knew if I was weak, they would be weak. If I was strong, they would be strong. I adapted and kept pushing ahead. We grew during this time when other solar companies were shutting down and had our best year yet as far as revenue numbers go.

After a few months, I was still doing lots of treatment and herbs on top of the plan for post-SOT treatment and keeping up with all my other habits. I was still doing hyperthermia, all my supplements, some medications, thyroid, testosterone, and injecting NAD subcutaneously for cellular repair and sermorelin injections at night to boost human growth hormone.

One day, I was reading a book, and my brain lit up.

We've all had the experience of reading a really engaging book when the content causes all cylinders in your brain to fire and form new connections and ideas. The dopamine will hit hard and make it difficult to put the book down. I had lost that since I had Lyme. For years, I couldn't read a book and have that feeling. My understanding of what I was reading was pretty low because of Lyme and brain fog. I would read them and pull out certain things and just act on them—surface-level thinking. I wasn't engaging my whole brain. I had forgotten what that felt like, and it felt good.

This experience confirmed that slowly but surely, the SOT treatment was doing something on a deeper level, a more lasting level, and I liked it. I was still staying neutral, and while I was getting better, I didn't want to say anything to jinx it. But I knew changes had taken hold.

Lyme puts a fog over not just your brain but your eyes. You tend to trust people too much or not see certain patterns. Lyme disconnects us from everything and everyone. But once your Lyme starts going away, you can feel connection again. Now, I felt better able to connect to people. I also was able to see red flags in people.

The robotic and survival-type feelings I had become accustomed to became more of an energizing feeling. When you have more vibrancy in your being, people become more interesting and exciting.

I started to feel emotions again. Regular emotions. The need to connect. I felt some actual joy and some emotions that are impossible to describe. These were actual feelings filling up my body like those of an eight-year-old waking up on Christmas Day.

People say you can practice gratitude, but that's for healthy people. When you are sick beyond reason, there is no such thing as gratitude; there is only survival. Now, I started feeling grateful for certain days when I felt good.

The improvement was fleeting, and I still had down days, but I was getting little glimpses, little mini-Christmases every now and then where I didn't feel like pure shit. My overall "stock graph" of my health was going up.

CHAPTER
19

"There will be painful moments in your life that will change your entire world in a matter of minutes. These moments will change you. Let them make you stronger, smarter, and kinder. But don't you go and become someone that you're not. Cry. Scream if you have to. Then straighten out that crown and keep moving."

—ERIN VAN VUREN

I BEGAN TO LET MY AMBITION RUN A LITTLE BIT AS I gained more confidence in the truth of my healing journey. I wanted to invest in real estate, so late in 2020, I spent at least thirty minutes every night going through a course in commercial real estate investing on Udemy, recommended by my friend Alan, while also listening to real estate audiobooks in my car. I wanted to be educated enough to make good decisions. Then, with the help of my friend Gavin in Utah, I bought two fourplexes there. That was a huge step for me in terms of realizing a personal goal and showing myself that I was on the road back to the old TJ.

Shortly after I bought my properties, in December 2020, I got hit with COVID-19, and it *demolished* me. I couldn't run the sales meetings, and a handful of other people on my team got it too. I thought the business was going to be in a dire situation. If we couldn't run the meetings and help guide people, we weren't in business.

At one point, I had such bad nerve pain I couldn't even do payroll. Pain shot down my legs. I could barely walk. I tried to massage the agony out, but it was nerve pain, so rubbing the muscles did nothing. Sitting down created an angle in my legs that caused ridiculous torture, and I couldn't think straight. It was only when I took Rick Simpson Oil, a marijuana oil, that I could actually look at my screen and complete payroll.

One night, I was so sick that I ordered a Bible from Amazon. I'm not really religious, so ordering a Bible late at night meant that I was either extremely sick and contemplating the end of my life, high from the Rick Simpson Oil, or both.

My isolation and depression during that illness deepened. My thoughts went dark. I saw how my business was flawed. I realized one of the sales managers needed to be fired and how that was going to be a wild ride. I hadn't done a good job of developing people so that if I was out of commission the business could function and still grow without me. It was purely dependent on me, which created enormous stress. Once the virus hit, I had the space to see all the changes I needed to make.

I also realized that I needed friends and support outside of the business. I needed to take care of me. I started researching groups and joined one.

I seriously contemplated whether or not I would be satisfied with my life if I died at this point. The one thing that came up was it would suck to die without having written a book. I resolved to write this book, and now you are reading it, all because of COVID.

To get over COVID I started getting vitamin IVs again. I already had hydroxychloroquine on hand from taking it previously for a Lyme coinfection, so I started taking that too. I also took some extra zinc and ramped up my elderberry usage. My lungs felt heavy, and I was short of breath. Thanks to a tip from a fellow Lyme warrior, I got ahold of liquid glutathione. I nebulized the glutathione and breathed it into my lungs daily. After two days my lungs felt almost back to normal.

The sales meetings I ran in December were super punishing. Later, after one of my sales reps had battled COVID, he said, "Shout out to you, dude. I feel like shit. I can't do anything."

"Yeah," I said. "I run sales meetings feeling worse than you do now."

I didn't want to be condescending, but it was a moment of connection. He understood that having Lyme isn't like having a cold. I may look fine on the outside, but it is agony on the inside. He was wiped out and in bed for four or five days, and I had been wiped out and trying to simultaneously build a business for years.

It took a long time to start feeling better after COVID, and the business got all messed up in the process. I was tired for a good three months. Everybody stopped working during the quarantine period when reps were sick because we couldn't knock doors, and there were no regular meetings to help keep the team going.

When I returned after two weeks, the first meeting I ran I had to sit down for the first half of it before standing up. It was annoying. I felt my Lyme had almost been in remission and I had bundles of energy before I got knocked all the way back down. I slowly had to build my way back up again.

It's hard falling down like that.

As I got better from COVID, a few times I actually felt good during the meetings. In one meeting I didn't feel sick at all. I was hitting the team hard with good motivation. I looked out at everyone in the room and thought, *Wow, this is so easy.* I had been so used to feeling like pure garbage.

* * *

As 2021 progressed, I had more ups and downs. I began microdosing mushrooms twice a week to see if it could produce neurogenesis in my brain. I tried microdosing LSD, but it wasn't my favorite because it made me lazy. In March, Dr. Hartzmann thought I still needed to knock a few of the coinfections out, so I started a combination of hydroxychloroquine and azithromycin. A few days later, as if it was magic, all of a sudden I felt the best I had felt since contracting Lyme. I took a ride on my mountain bike. I did a pushup competition and didn't get messed up after. I was selling deals almost like I used to, selling twenty personal deals in two months while running the company. I was having spiritual experiences and feelings. I was feeling gratitude to be alive, the sunset looked amazing, and I thought I had made it.

Maybe that Lyme SOT cured me!

This lasted for about a month and a half.

Then I woke up one day and I felt *horrible*. I felt even worse than before I started the hydroxychloroquine and azithromycin combo. Now I didn't know what to do.

I tried more SOTs, three in total. One for Bartonella and two for HSV. None of them worked. The Lyme SOT in March helped, but the three others afterward didn't do anything for me. I started getting so bad again I began thinking it wasn't worth it. I wanted to die. My brain was trying to figure out how to cope with the pain by ending it. I was alone in my house, isolated, running the business with the responsibility of it all, the walls crashing in on me, dealing with betrayal, deceit, people trying to steal my reps, not knowing who I could trust. I could barely breathe from the stress and health problems.

I quickly booked a ketamine and NAD (nicotinamide adenine dinucleotide) IV for mid-May. When I got in there I was hanging on by a thread. I got in there just in time before ending it all. There was so much NAD in the IV, the price was almost $2,000, but I didn't care. The IV took three hours.

While under the influence, I worked through a lot of emotional stuff I was holding in. The ketamine set me free. I saw visuals, I traveled around, it showed me my weak points, and finally, I was able to relax. The relaxation part and forgetting about the world let me open up to myself. To stop compartmentalizing to survive my health trauma so I could keep the business going. I felt it all.

After that, I changed my view on ketamine. I saw its therapeutic potential. I did it a few more times, but one time there was too much ketamine, and I forgot I existed. I went into the blackest of the black. I was flying around space like I was in the movie *Interstellar*. I saw a glass container with coffins inside and was lowered inside one, the coffin door closing, and I experienced ego death. After the coffin door closed, I saw my dead grandfather, brother, and two friends Spencer and Carlos. I tried to make out Spencer's face but couldn't see it fully. The ketamine told me, "Isn't that sad...as time goes on, the memory fades...That's why people are so important." I felt I needed to create a family and have children.

When I finally came out of it, I started crying because I was back to the world. I let the IV person know to not give me that dosage ever again.

* * *

I had known about Bee Venom Therapy for a long time. It just seemed so extreme. But then again, wouldn't that make me a hypocrite if I always talked about doing whatever it takes to succeed but I was too closed-minded to doing some bee stings?

So I ordered some bees. Someone I met through Facebook walked me through the whole process: where to buy the right tweezers, where to order the bees, and how to catch one and sting myself. You are supposed to start with one sting and gradually make your way up to stinging yourself ten times three times per week.

I would open the container a little bit to let one bee fly out, spray her with water so she couldn't fly, grab her leg with straight tweezers, then use angled tweezers to grab her right in the midsection. Then I would place her against my back, an inch away from my spine. The bee would sting, which actually doesn't hurt that bad, there is just a burning sensation afterwards.

The only thing I didn't really like about it is that it feels a bit creepy, but whatever. The stings actually helped me with my symptoms. Every time I tried to get to two bee stings, I would get chills and fever like I was getting a cold or flu and I had to go back to one sting. I had enough bees for three weeks. I ordered more, but they died in the Nevada heat during shipping.

I was referred to someone in San Diego that said she got into Lyme remission using a chlorine dioxide solution. Some people know it by "Miracle Mineral Solution" or MMS. I tried drinking that for a few days, but it made my stomach feel weird, and I was a bit off, so I stopped. It also tastes like you are drinking pool water, which isn't exactly pleasant.

At the same time, someone referred me to a health specialist in the UK who said the main thing I had to look at was autoimmunity. They ran some tests and started me on a strict diet, avoiding all sorts of foods that can react with EBV.

I felt good again.

For about two months, I kicked ass. I was selling multiple deals while running the business because I couldn't help myself. I hired a new person as head of sales. I started a call center in Mexico. I was on fire, and I loved it. I pushed myself too hard, though, and my health took a dip.

Once I had energy, I realized just how angry I was. I hadn't let myself expend emotional energy on being angry when I was sick, because that just wiped me out. Now I was angry at the people that screwed me over. Angry that I can't exercise. Angry that I have to throttle myself. Angry that I can't really travel. Angry that I can't truly be myself. Angry that I feel like shit all the time. Angry and about to prove to the world just what I could actually do when I wasn't sick, since they were used to the 30 percent TJ. And angry about all the lost time and at how much I wanted to do.

* * *

In late 2021, I went on peptides. I started taking BPC-157, LL-37, Thymosin Alpha-1, and Thymosin Beta-4. I heard a doctor in Los Angeles talk about peptides and how they can help the immune system finally take care of Lyme disease. You can kill it off as much as you want, but without getting your immune system to function properly so it can handle Lyme on its own, you'll never truly have your health back.

The BPC-157 helps heal tissues. LL-37 kills pathogens. Thymosin Beta-4 is intended to increase Th1/Treg and reduce Th2/Th17, along with providing additional rejuvenating properties. If that sounds confusing, basically the goal is to help shift the immune system to more intracellular action to get at the Lyme, since Lyme hides in the body. Thymosin Alpha-1 is to help boost immune function, similar to Thymosin Beta-4.

Within a week of starting these peptides, I began feeling better. I had energy and enthusiasm and was feeling a wide range of positive emotions. I started dating someone in Los Angeles. *Oh, this is it! I found the key!* Then after Christmas, I got COVID again and BOOM, back to feeling like shit again. *Son of a bitch!*

In early 2022 a few major things happened for me.

First, I booked myself for a week into The Raj, an Ayurvedic health center in Fairfield, Iowa. I had heard that the Panchakarma treatment there could really help with Lyme.

Just before going to Fairfield, I was connected to a mold specialist, Dr. Rudbeck. This was the second big thing. I had been through many, many tests, but I had never been tested for mold toxicity. I did urine testing with RealTime Laboratories that showed high numbers of multiple toxic mycotoxins in my body.

This was significant because I have been treating and treating and treating for all kinds of things, but never for toxic mold, which can be just as bad as Lyme. Dr. Rudbeck said I probably had elevated toxic mold levels going all the way back to 2017. I needed to fix the mold problem, which was causing inflammation, before I was going to be able to get better. Also, mold interferes with thiamin absorption, which had a lot to do with my low energy and depression.

There are three steps to mold treatment. First, I had to make sure I was not living in a moldy environment. So long as I lived with mold, I was not going to be able to defeat mold. I tested my house and found that no mycotoxins from my house were present in my urine, so I didn't need to pack up and move. Second, I needed to take the correct binders, in the correct order and pacing, to pull mold out of my body. If I tried to push too hard on this step I could end up feeling worse and having to back off.

Third, I had to take antifungal medications to eradicate the mold that had infected me (mold usually prefers the gut or the sinuses, and I recently had a staph infection in my nose).

On top of that, I was going to take supplements thirty minutes before eating each meal, since I was having mast cell reactions to foods, and that's why I hated eating so much. I would take quercetin, histamine digest, and perimine thirty minutes before each meal, and take quercetin before bed every night to help calm the mast cell reaction down. A lot of my symptoms were supposedly from histamine/mast cell problems.

The mold infections I suffered from were getting in the way of my understanding whether I was treating the Lyme, Bartonella, and other tick-borne infections correctly. Even if I had the right approach, it wouldn't work, or wouldn't work very well, so long as the mold was active. Once I got the mold out, I could focus on the Lyme. Paying attention to my symptoms, Dr. Rudbeck said, would be as effective a way as any other for me to know how well my Lyme treatment was progressing.

* * *

This was amazing information to get before I started the Panchakarma retreat, and I made an appointment to start treatment to help detox further, called the Patricia Kane protocol, as soon as I got home.

Panchakarma is an Ayurvedic treatment modality to get waste and toxins out of the body. It involves a few main treatments: cleansing of the five sense organs and nervous system through the nasal system; cleansing the digestive system through improved digestive function; cleansing the intestines through purgation; cleansing the colon through enemas; and lots and lots of oil massages. There are also stages of preparation and recovery.

As with almost all my treatments, I did this because someone recommended it. My friend Jeff's wife, Sarah, is a doctor who has battled Lyme disease and mold herself, and she said Panchakarma was a real turning point for her. That was a powerful endorsement.

This experience was a first for me. I had done a lot of things to recover my health, but I had never taken a week off from my business and set my phone on Do Not Disturb. That week in February 2022 was a week for Taylor and TJ to get reacquainted, but this time in a peaceful setting.

The biggest thing I saw at The Raj was that everyone was happy and glowing and had energy. (Seriously, even all the old people.) I started asking what they were doing differently, and every single person said "meditation." They were sitting and meditating for at least twenty minutes twice a day.

The treatments were useful, but the most important thing that happened to me in Fairfield was mental. One of the big things they promote in Fairfield is that you have to recharge in order to be effective in life. In order to be efficient in the external world, you have to be efficient in the internal world. I began to meditate more and more seriously.

One day in Iowa, lying in the clinic getting a treatment, I had a powerful moment. I asked myself, *Why am I sick? How am I contributing to staying sick?*

It was such a powerful question.

Once I asked the question, I kept asking it. I was three and a half years into my business, almost six years into my Lyme journey, and I had never taken this kind of time for myself. The questions kept coming: *What role do I have in my illness? Where did I go wrong? Are there any blind spots?*

Since then, I've meditated twice a day to seek those answers. I am on my journey to what I believe to be the last missing piece of this puzzle for me.

I understand that the universe delivers lessons. Some practices say that the universe delivers exactly the lesson you need. Sometimes I find myself asking, "Alright, universe, have I learned this lesson yet? What else do I need to learn? Because, wow, I feel I've had enough."

When I returned home, I did my first session of the Patricia Kane protocol, which I did from 9:00 a.m. to 2:00 p.m., Tuesdays and Fridays. It included both IVs and colonics, sometimes at the same time. The first time I went through the Patricia Kane treatment my hands were shaking, my heart was racing, my whole body was freaking out, and I didn't feel good. I was determined to give it a chance to work. Then one day, all of a sudden, I just started getting energy again.

The Patricia Kane protocol is centered on doing IVs of phosphatidylcholine, sodium phenylbutyrate, glutathione, and folinic acid; doing methylcobalamin injections; and increasing your intake of essential fatty acids to heal your gut and heal yourself at the cellular level.

As I continued my mold detoxing protocol, I started waking up feeling energized, I started feeling motivated again, I started feeling enthusiastic. This time, I am confident I am not on the hope roller coaster. This time, I am confident that the ladder is not about to fall over. This time, I still have my feet on the ground.

* * *

It is only a matter of time before I get to 90 percent-plus. Over the last five years, it has been one hellish roller coaster ride, but if you look at it like a stock graph, there have been plenty of ups and downs, and the overall trend is up.

I believe that a lot of people who don't recover from Lyme for a long period of time are missing major pieces like I was. Now that I'm cranking away at all these elements, detoxing the mold and adjusting my mindset, I'm confident that my immune system will begin working properly.

I realized when I was meditating that I had to make a commitment to what's best for me despite all the pressures of the outside world. I have to trust that commitment as a compass. I had been living a pattern where I was doing well, but then things got crazy at work, and I couldn't take time to take care of myself, and I started to regress in my health. For so long my brain was wired to push, push, push, feeling that everyone is out for themselves, business is cutthroat, and life boils down to fight or die.

There is another path. I see now that the opposite behavior is that I have to surrender. I have to have kindness toward myself. Gentleness toward myself. I have to go slow where I used to go fast and never stop. I am starting to see that I sometimes have to place my well-being above the business, to have stronger boundaries, and to truly heal myself in all areas.

It's hard for me to make that transition. It's hard for me to unlearn the type A behavior that is so deeply wired into my sense of self. I'm not quite there, but I am trying to balance these things.

EPILOGUE

HAVING SEVERE HEALTH ISSUES IS ONE OF THE HARDEST things I've endured. Yet I can't deny the gifts that come with it.

The hardest part of having a chronic illness is that you can't live the life you want. The one you used to live. You used to have the energy to exercise, eat anything, travel, and do whatever you wanted to do. All of that used to make up who you were—someone who no longer exists. That experience is why, when you do win, you will kick life's ass. If you can survive all the suffering, fatigue, and bullshit and not give up, then nothing difficult in a normal life will ever stop you.

The harsh truth is on the one end, being this sick is the worst suffering you can imagine. But on the other end, you'll come out much stronger and everything will be that much more beautiful.

We want the pain to end now, but it won't. It will take time, but life can improve. That is the key. The only way to get through it is to continue on until one day you find that relief. One year of suffering can feel like ten years of suffering. You will undergo lots of pain tolerance and pain compartmentalization training.

Humans don't define themselves by their happy moments. We yearn for them, but typically don't define ourselves by joy and the good things that have happened. We define ourselves by the hardships we have overcome.

Healing Lyme is like hiking Mount Everest solo. Sometimes you climb mountains with a group; other times, people climb Mount Everest alone. The lessons you learn hiking alone are different than what you would learn in a group. Lyme is known as the "do it yourself disease." As I suffered in loneliness, I started to see that purpose and meaning are bigger than materialism, that people and friends are more important than anything, and that health is the greatest gift.

Experiences like Lyme teach you a lot about life. You learn a lot about yourself, going on rides straight to the depths of hell. I learned that when you have a health issue, you have to flow with the river and accept it. It was one of the harder things for me to come to grips with. I learned it is hard to judge people in dire situations with health conditions or mental health problems.

One of the hardest things to learn has been that I have to take care of myself first. You might think that's an odd thing to read, after everything you've read about all the things I did to try to heal. But this is different. What I've had trouble learning is that I have to put myself and my health first. Not my business. Not the people I am trying to help. Not the deals I am trying to make.

* * *

Please understand that you have to make hard decisions to heal. A lot of times, that means saying no. This was incredibly difficult for me, because I drive myself so hard, and I am so focused on performance.

When you are faced with an opportunity, such as a job to make a lot of money, and every fiber of your being wants it, your ego wants it, you know you could do it before Lyme, you have pressure from people and friends...you have to accept the truth. You just...can't...take it right now. Going that hard could set you back. Nobody who has ever been in the deep end of Lyme would risk anything that would put them back into such an agonizing space. So you learn how to say no. As you've read, it took me a long time to learn that lesson fully and accept the reality of my situation. But I had to learn it. And I'm still learning it.

You have to say no to a lot of things. Your life becomes more restricted. You see fewer people. You do less. You focus more on yourself. This is essential because that is how you are going to get better. The deeper I went, the more I realized I needed to rely on principles and values. My principles, as I described, revolved around focusing on other people rather than myself.

You can wake up in the middle of the night with your heart beating rapidly and barely able to move, thinking about checking yourself into the hospital even though you know that won't do anything. That's how scared you are. You'll lie in the bathtub for an hour exhausted. You'll have no appetite and have to force yourself to eat because you know you need to.

Sometimes you have to cry a bit to let it out. Sometimes, you suffer in silence because you can't let people know what's really going on.

Saying no might look selfish to others. It might look like you are only out for yourself. But you have no other choice. You have to make it to the peak of Everest and back. Although the outside world might not understand, you know the choice you need to make. If you take that other route up the mountain, you'll fall and freeze in a ridge, even though everyone else is telling you to go that way. You have to go your way. So you do.

* * *

I developed a lot of adaptations to survive and to get through Lyme. When I look back at how often I thought about killing myself, and how many times I tried, or at least tried to try, I'm amazed I made it this far. I kept playing tricks on my brain and making deals with myself. I'd give myself a suicide carrot, saying, "OK, if we don't feel better by X date, then I'll kill myself." My brain needed an exit. It needed to know we weren't going to suffer like this for fifty years.

When I think about why I didn't go through with it, I believe it was because there was always one tiny piece of my brain that had a compelling argument. It said to me, "If you kill yourself, it's over. You're dead. But if there's even a 2 percent chance that you'll get better, you still have that chance."

Think about those odds. Two percent doesn't sound like much, but when I was knocking on doors, making bank, and breaking down my self-limiting beliefs about what I was capable of, I was only working on 1 percent odds. I had to knock one hundred doors to make a sale. Those are 1 percent odds. Two percent odds looked good enough for me to keep going.

If you're in a space like that, step back. You don't know what your life will become. In 2017, 2018, and 2019, I could not imagine that I would have written a book or be running a multimillion-dollar business with more than forty people working for the company. I am looking forward now to starting a family. I never could have imagined that then. In a few years, you might be living your best life ever. You simply can't know. You might be ill and suffering now, and you might still be in a few years. But you might not, too, and you have to play that chance.

Suicidal thoughts are a warning—they're like a "check engine" light on your dashboard. Because of the shame around suicide, too many people who have those thoughts keep them to themselves—often until it's too late. That's much more dangerous than talking about them. If you have Lyme, suicidal thoughts can be a symptom. They can be your brain trying to protect you. That may seem paradoxical, but the brain's job is to protect you. If all you have is unrelenting pain, the brain may, in a twisted way, convince itself that you will get out of the pain by killing yourself.

If you have suicidal thoughts, step back from them and ask, "Oh, shit—what is this telling me? What's going on? What do I need?" Get curious about the thoughts themselves, rather than taking them seriously. And talk to somebody about them. Seriously.

Lyme showed me that I didn't know how to love myself. Nobody taught me. I had to learn that, so I created Taylor and TJ to teach me. I didn't know what I was doing at the time, but that's what they did. You might be in a similar situation now. You might have lost the things you love that you once used to define yourself. You might have seen yourself as a marathon runner. Or a good mom. Or a successful businesswoman. Lyme might have taken all that away. If it did, or it does, what will you see? What will be left? You may have to look into the abyss of yourself.

You can do it. You can look in there and see someone to love. In fact, you have to do it.

* * *

I succeeded in my Lyme journey for many reasons. I put high pain tolerance and an almost spiritual level of willpower near the top of the list. You can tolerate more pain than you realize. And you can do more than you may think you can. You may tell yourself, "I just can't do X," but if you had a child with you, and the child would die if you didn't do X, you'd do X. There would be no question. You can embrace that mentality. When I didn't have the energy to do what I had to do at work, sometimes I would grab Carlos's dog tag and tell myself, "You have to do this." I viewed the success of my business as a life-and-death matter. There was no other choice.

Sometimes I undertook desperate measures—an injection of Toradol, a mushroom microdose, a quick IV to get a boost and keep going to do what I had to do before I could lie down and rest. I would tell myself, "All you've got to do is survive, be on your game for an hour and a half, and then you can rest."

I had my tools, and I knew how to negotiate with myself.

However...I probably took it too far. I pushed myself so hard for so long that I wore myself out. I didn't let my immune system recover. I have tried to learn that I don't actually need to be so hardcore. That I should take one day off a week. I don't need to go out and knock doors to close deals when my body is broken down; I can sell one less deal and have my body get better. I have to learn that, even though I am super type A, the best thing I can do is prioritize getting healthy. I can be a bit less type A.

It's been incredibly hard for me to say, "I can't." I have told myself a story for a long time that the reason my business has succeeded is because of me alone and because of my willingness to support and help the people who work with me. I have told myself the story that the only way people will care about me, want to be around me, love me is if I "produce" in some way. I have to accept that is not true, or not as true as it once might have been.

I learned this the hard way. Earlier in this book, I described how I see myself as a Lamborghini limited to driving twenty-five miles per hour, even though I know I could go 140, and I want to go 140. I learned this lesson by repeatedly driving my car too hard and breaking it. Again and again. I finally realized I should stop breaking the car.

* * *

You might be thinking at this point, "Well shit, TJ, you basically wrote a whole long story about how shitty your experience has been, your ups and downs, and all the wild stuff you went through—but what am I supposed to do?" I can't say I have an exact answer. Why? Because every person is so different. But if I was going to start over, here's what I would do.

Check Your Mindset

I believe that every problem has a solution. If what I was doing wasn't working, that just meant I hadn't found the solution yet. I have to keep going, keep hacking away. Every time I failed was a new lesson. Every failed treatment is one step closer to the treatment that will work. I told myself I had to play a long game; this might take many years.

Get the Best Team

I would find one of the top doctors in the world on Lyme, and I would find one of the leading people on the immune system and work with both of them. I would grab the book *New Paradigms in Lyme Disease Treatment* by Connie Strasheim, and go through it to hear from some of the top doctors for Lyme treatment modalities and reach out to the ones you resonate with. I would get a very comprehensive test of my Lyme, coinfections, and immune system to rule out autoimmune issues or other things like mold that might be holding me back.

Partner with Your Doctors

Help your medical team do the best work they can. That means more than keeping your records organized. It also means recognizing that 80 percent of your healing depends on you. I talked to one woman suffering from Lyme who said she couldn't get better—but she also couldn't give up her addiction to Burger King. No wonder she couldn't get better; she wasn't willing to do her part.

When you are working with anyone in the medical profession, try to make it as easy as possible for them to help you. Use my system of health folders. Be meticulous and organized about tracking your health history, lab results, medications, and protocols. Unless you're fully engaged, they are going to miss things that they should be aware of. You are not putting yourself in their hands; you are partnering with them. You need to work together toward solutions.

When it came to finding doctors to work with, I relied on referrals. If I heard that a particular doctor had helped other people like me, I looked them up. This is where it's so important to have a support network. However you can find a group, do it. Lyme can make you feel lonely and isolated. Not only is that depressing, it's flat-out bad for your health. Make the effort to connect with other Lyme sufferers and those who work with them. Yes, there will be bad apples, but the vast majority will be people who genuinely want to help you, even if that means doing no more than listening to you.

Be Open to Treatment

If your infections are really, really bad, then medications and antibiotics might be necessary for a while. For instance, Coartem changed my brain fog permanently. Some people are against antibiotics; others are for antibiotics. What's right for you will depend on your situation.

Do What's Most Important First, and Adjust

There is an order of operations to this. It doesn't make sense to go after viruses if you have active Lyme and mold, since the Lyme and mold need to be handled first for the immune system to have any breathing room. If you don't handle the most immune-taxing problems first, you'll be fighting an uphill battle.

I would pick the top thing you can do and do that for a while, then pivot if needed. Lyme is complex, and each person has a different makeup of what is happening, but the good news is that if something doesn't work you have ten backup plans to try.

The top things that I have done for myself are these:

- Hyperthermia (both in clinic and at home)

- Specific antibiotic treatments

- Diet and herbal supplements

- Getting my hormones in check

- Detox methods

- Gut healing

- Peptides

- Lyme SOT

- Limbic system retraining

Support Your Body

I would get a method to help bring the pathogen level down while taking probiotics and protecting my gut; work on gut repair; simultaneously and religiously do detox (such as detox baths, saunas, etc.); take at least a walk every day for exercise; focus on getting excellent sleep; and then dial in my diet with testing and experimentation to eat in a way that doesn't cause inflammation.

Get Mental Health Help

I would get a therapist or someone that can help me cope with the mental health aspect of Lyme, preferably one that has had Lyme or a serious health condition themselves. You know my mental health has been bad. It's really, really hard to cope emotionally and mentally with being held back, not to mention the fact that these infections actually go in the brain and cause personality issues, rage, depression, bipolar disorder, etc. The biggest thing I lacked was support and community. Isolation hurts your immune system.

Don't Overdo Supplements

"More is not always better." Several doctors told me that. I should have been more strategic with supplements instead of throwing everything at the Lyme. I take fewer supplements now, more targeted. Take the top ones, and don't overload your system.

Understand How and When Different Treatments Will Help

Stem cells were alright, but not a cure, and I came at them wrong. They have their place to repair the body, but their real role comes later, once you are already on the up, and they can help repair the damage as you improve. Otherwise, you are just putting a Band-Aid on a body that's going to get wrecked from the pathogens. Until I got the mold and Lyme-induced active damage to my body down, stem cells just weren't going to be able to be their most effective.

Put Yourself First

There is still a part of me that has a really hard time putting myself first. I may need a rest day, but the demands of my business are never-ending. No matter what I do, there is always more to be done. People always want more from me. I keep trying to prioritize my health journey, to accept that it's OK if my business suffers a little bit. That's an ongoing struggle for me.

I'm wired to produce in business. I just am. Even when my body is screaming at me to slow down, I am like a racehorse that just wants to run. I have had to learn—I am continuing to learn—that my life now is the way it is. That I face a reality that is different from what I want. That I have to surrender to that in order to improve.

On all levels, I am a lot better than I used to be. As I write this book, my company has forty-two people and does $3.2 million in revenue. I have a long-term vision of having eight or ten offices around the country, each with fifteen or twenty sales reps. Life is a lot easier. My down days now are way better than my best days a few years ago. I feel I've made progress up Maslow's hierarchy of needs to where I can focus on self-actualizing. I've survived a lot, I've done a lot, now I really want to hit my potential in terms of what kind of impact I can make in this lifetime.

I could not have thought that way a couple of years ago.

All the different things I did, I did because I was searching for ways to feel better and to heal myself. Many did not help. Some of them might even have done some damage. But eventually, I found what worked for me. When I think about how I got better, it's not about this protocol or that treatment, it's about the mindset I had to keep pushing forward no matter what. I negotiated with myself to stay alive at certain points, and I never stopped trying to get better.

There was a time when I was really angry about the things Lyme took away from me: traveling, going out to dinner or drinks with friends, dating easily, working out. None of those have come back into my life yet. I still have some anger from time to time. But what has come back is my ability to work and to make an impact on the people around me. That has become incredibly valuable. I try to focus not so much now on what I don't have; I think about what I do have and what I can do with it.

There is a spiritual component to pushing forward. Lyme has shown me that I have a deeper reservoir, call it spirit or soul or life force, that wants to be on this planet and make a difference. I didn't realize the depth of that deeper reservoir until I reckoned with the darkness of Lyme.

My life is different now because it is functional. I am not cured of Lyme. Am I 100 percent? No. I'm still searching for ways to build on my improvements. I know that if I can get the pathogen load lower and increase the capacity of my body to handle what's going on, I should be able to contain the Lyme and coinfections and live a healthy life. We all have viruses or pathogens in us, whether it is smallpox or EBV, that are in us forever. I am still searching for answers to get better and better.

I've come a long way. And I don't plan on stopping until I get to 90 percent-plus of where I was pre-Lyme. I'm the wild person that will try anything, and I hope my journey gives you some insight on potential paths you can take and that you can get better.

I am so much better than I used to be. My journey was hard, and when I look back I can see that in some ways I made it harder than it needed to be. The payoff is sweet. Not only do I feel better, not only am I returning to my old self, but I have a newfound understanding of what matters in life, and I have the ability to help you. I hope you learn from my journey. I hope you are inspired to take action to restore your health. I hope you find just one thing in this book that helps you.

APPENDICES

MY SUPPLEMENTS & EXPERIENCES WITH THEM THROUGH MY LYME JOURNEY

Note—Keep in mind for some supplements, I may not have known if they helped or not individually because I took so much stuff at once, but the combination of supplements together often was helping me when I couldn't isolate the improvement down to one single supplement.

5-HTP: Amino acid to help boost serotonin and feel better, as well as potentially help me sleep. Gave me weird effects, didn't make me feel better or worse, but loopier.

5-MTHF 5 mg (Thorne): Methyl form of a B vitamin, supposed to help with my genetic mutation and get over Lyme. This could have made me worse, actually.

ADR Formula: Supposed to help give the adrenal glands a boost to have more energy and help for my body to fight off the disease. No idea if it helped or not.

Adrenal Support Plus: Supposed to help with my cortisol dip around noon in supporting the adrenal glands, hoping to gain more stable energy. I am not sure if they are helping or not, although I am seeing improvement on the entire supplement protocol I am currently taking, which includes this supplement.

Allergy Research Free Aminos: Amino acids are to give me the necessary building blocks to produce neurotransmitters and for overall health. Goal was to feel better energy-wise and mentally. I feel like this helps, but I cannot say for sure.

Alpha-Lipoic Acid: Supposed to help boost glutathione (which would help my body's immune system fight off Lyme) and reduce inflammation caused by Lyme. I am not sure if it helped or not, but in combination with everything else it has.

Astaxanthin: Antioxidant, supposed to protect cells from damage and improve the immune system. I am not sure if it helped or not.

Astragalus: Supposed to regulate the immune system so it reacts better to the Lyme pathogen and does not cause as much inflammation. I am not sure if it worked or not.

Banderol: Goal was to reduce Lyme. It has helped me fight Lyme, and I still take it. I have taken it for years to put constant pressure on the Lyme bacterium. It has helped me a lot. (Banderol,

Samento, Houttuynia, Mora, Cumanda, and Burbur Pinella are all part of the Cowden protocol, and NutraMedix is a brand that makes a lot of those.)

Beta-Sitosterol: Was supposed to help my hormones and libido. I noticed a short-term increase in libido, but not long-term.

Betaine Plus HP: Supposed to help with digestion, as betaine helps break food down. Can't say if it worked or not.

BioAstin: Supposed to reduce inflammation, which would help me feel better. I have no idea if it helped or not.

Bio-C Plus 1000: Vitamin C supplement; see also Bio-FCTS and C-Salts Buffered Vitamin C.

Biocidin: Taken to break up the biofilm that Lyme and coinfections hide in to avoid detection from the immune system. I feel like this helped, although I did not take it long-term.

Bio-FCTS: Vitamin C with quercetin, to help with inflammatory response. Not sure if it helped.

Bio-Immunozyme Forte: Supposed to help support the immune system and have an antioxidant effect. I have no idea if it helped or not.

BodyBio Balance Oil: Fatty oil to help balance my fatty acid composition based on my lab work. At the core level, cells are made up of fats and have fatty acid walls, and with a proper balance they can become healthy. I feel like this has helped.

BodyBio Calcium Magnesium Butyrate: Butyrate is produced by your gut microbes and has many important functions within the human body, particularly for digestive health, supporting brain health, and protecting against disease. Supposed to help heal my gut. I have a feeling this has helped, but I cannot say for sure.

BodyBio Evening Primrose Oil: Fatty oil to help balance my fatty acid composition based on my lab work. At the core level, cells are made up of fats and have fatty acid walls, and with a proper balance they can become healthy. I feel like this has helped.

BodyBio PC: Phosphatidylcholine is a fatty acid that is a component of cell membranes. Due to immune-mediated and direct damage from Lyme disease, cell membranes throughout the body—including nerves—become damaged. I take this in an IV and as a supplement. The goal was to help my stomach heal and to feel better. PC has been helping me a lot. My appetite has also been coming back.

BPC-157: Helps heal tissues and the body. Was using it to help heal my gut, and that helps with immune system and everything. I feel like this has helped.

Burbur-Pinella (NutraMedix): Help the brain and nerves, supposed to detox and help the body. I still take it and have taken it for a very long time. I would say this has helped me.

CBD: Hoping it would help with sleep, curb inflammation, help with pain. I took the liquid CBD and CBD patches on my back. The liquid CBD would help me sleep. If I was awake or knew I was going to have a hard time falling asleep, I would take a bunch, and it would help. I would put a patch on my back if I was feeling a lot of Lyme symptoms, and it would help curb the pain. CBD is always in my back pocket to use when I need it.

Chelated Zinc: Zinc supposedly boosts the immune system, which would in turn help me fight off the Lyme and therefore feel better. I can't say whether or not this had a definitive effect.

Chinese Skullcap: Used for anti-inflammatory effects. Supposed to help ease the symptoms. I am not sure if it helped or not.

Choline (Standard Process): Lab work showed I was deficient in choline, so I took the supplement for a while. I cannot say if it made me feel better since I started too many supplements at the same time.

ChromeMate GTF 600 (Pure Encapsulations): My lab work showed I was deficient in Chromium, so I took this supplement for a while. Can't say if it helped me or not, I just knew that I needed it.

Cilantro: Used for detox to help get the bad stuff out of my body. Since I have taken a lot of things to kill the Lyme, I also need help in detox so the Herxheimer reaction isn't too crazy. I believe it has helped me, but I cannot say 100 percent.

ClearVite GLB (Apex): To help heal the stomach. Can't say for sure if it has helped, but I believe it is helping.

Collagen Peptides: Supposed to support joints and connective tissues. I have taken collagen for a long time because I read that Lyme likes to eat your joints, and I never wanted to end up in a wheelchair or similar. Can't say if it helped for sure or not.

Colloidal Silver Spray & Colloidal Silver Argentyn 23 Liquid: Supposed to help kill off bacterium and pathogens. I am not sure if it worked or not.

Colostrum: Supposed to help heal the gut and boost the immune system. I am not sure if it worked or not.

CoQ10: Antioxidant. Have taken it on and off for overall health effects. Cannot say for sure if it helped me.

Cordyceps Extract (Host Defense Mushrooms): Small amount of mushroom extract is supposed to help regulate the immune system so that it responds better to the pathogens and also doesn't overreact, causing a lot of symptoms. I cannot say if it helped me or not.

Cumanda: Antifungal, antiviral, antiparasitic, used for Lyme coinfections and Lyme itself. I noticed a dramatic effect when taking this. I believe it helped kill off/manage Bartonella. The Idaho doctor would have me take it when I had certain rashes, and I noticed with the effects that it was powerful. I would take it more than was recommended because I knew it helped me. Before my second stand-up comedy show it helped relieve my symptoms to the point where I was able to do one of the best performances I did during that time. It wasn't a cure-all, but it 100 percent had a noticeable effect for me.

Cytozyme-THY: Thymus concentrate to help boost the immune system; no idea if it helped or not.

Delta Sleep: Supposed to aid with deeper sleep over time. I hoped to have higher-quality sleep. I cannot say if it has helped.

DGL (Nature's Way): To help my stomach not be as inflamed when eating. It had some mild effect but no longer needed.

DHEA: Hormone produced in the adrenal gland which helps other hormones like testosterone. I have had lots of issues with my adrenal glands, fatigue, depression, low testosterone, etc. This 100 percent has a major impact. It gives me more energy and makes me feel way better. Whenever I try to get off it, I crash. It has helped me a lot.

Digestive Enzymes: This is taken before each meal and is supposed to help with digestion. I thought it would help me with eating, since that is often a painful and shitty experience. I am pretty sure it has helped. This is a very common supplement a lot of people know about. I have taken forms of digestive enzymes for a long time.

DLPA: Amino acid that results in an increased production of catecholamines/neurotransmitters for focus, as well as having an opioid effect. Would help me feel a bit better, but using it long-term made me feel worse.

Elderberry: My hope was it would help reduce viral load to decrease the effects of stuff like EBV. I don't take it anymore and have no idea if it had any effect.

EnteroVite (Apex): Short-chain fatty acids to help heal the gut. I believe this has helped. It has butyrate in it, which is one of the supplements I still take to this day that helps with my stomach.

Epithalon: Supposed to help with sleep and with reducing auto-immune disorder affecting the thyroid. I cannot say if it has helped.

Excellacor: This has a bunch of enzymes; I took it while doing hyperthermia. The goal was that the enzymes would help break everything up as I was heating up my body and hopefully killing stuff off. I am not sure if it helped or not.

GABA: An amino acid to help produce more of the neurotransmitter that creates a state of calm and reduces anxiety. Would take some at night to help sleep. It helped some but was not super powerful.

Garlic Extract: Supposed to be antimicrobial to kill stuff. Not sure if it helped or not.

GI Support: Powder with ingredients like glutamine, arabinogalactans, deglycyrrhizinated licorice, aloe vera leaf, slippery elm, marshmallow to help soothe the gut and heal the gut. Gut health is one of the most important things for your immune system, and antibiotics destroy the gut. My hope was that it would help with my stomach to improve my Lyme. Can't say 100 percent if it helped, but I would say there is an 85 percent chance.

Glucosamine: Supposed to help the joints. After seeing people that have Lyme ending up in wheelchairs, I was terrified of having my joints get messed up. (The doctor that diagnosed me in San Diego said I had tendinitis in my knees.) I took this for a long time. I have no idea if it helped.

Glutamine: Supposed to help heal the gut lining. This helped me over the years. I would notice fewer symptoms in my stomach, such as low appetite or pain while eating.

Glutathione Recycler (Apex): Goal is to help the synthesis and recycling of glutathione, which helps the immune system. I can't say for sure if it works but my guess is it is helping.

Goldenseal Root: Supposed to have antimicrobial and mild immune-stimulating effects. I have no idea if it helped.

Gut-Specific Fish Oil (Microbiome Labs): Fish oil to help with healthy fatty acids and overall well-being. Most likely caused an imbalance of Omega-3 in my body, which I am now working on balancing back.

H-PLR (Apex): Goal was to help the immune system and the gut/intestinal mucosal immunity. Can't say if it worked or not.

Houttuynia: Was supposed to help with coinfections, used in traditional Chinese medicine to treat various inflammatory and infectious diseases. I felt a reduction of symptoms from taking it (symptoms were all the usual fatigue, brain fog, depression, aches, etc.).

IAG: Arabinogalactans, which are supposed to help the immune system fight off infections. I have no idea if it helped enhance my natural killer cells or not while I was taking it.

iMagT Powder: Magnesium supplement taken at night to help me sleep. It has helped me stay asleep and sleep deeper, and having proper sleep is essential to feeling good and having the immune system be able to handle Lyme.

Innate GI Response: Supposed to help soothe and heal the gut. I have noticed that GI supplements I take in the morning contribute to my gut not being in pain, reduce bloating, etc. The better my gut has become, the more my appetite comes back as well.

Ion Gut Health: Supposed to help my gut heal. I don't know if it made a difference or not; my guess would be no.

Japanese Knotweed: One of the compounds in this plant is supposed to be effective against Lyme. Also supposed to enhance blood flow. I have taken it for a long time and believe that it has helped me heal.

Jigsaw Adrenal Cocktail: Supposed to help provide the adrenal glands with nutrients to function better. My adrenal glands have had a hard time from all the stress of my life and the massive stress of Lyme, as well as the body trying to fight off Lyme. I am not sure if it has helped but I feel like it has.

Keto DHEA: Hormone produced in the adrenal gland which helps other hormones like testosterone. I have had lots of issues with my adrenal glands, like fatigue, depression, low testosterone, etc. This 100 percent has a major impact. It gives me more energy and makes me feel way better. Whenever I try to get off it, I crash. Some people may benefit more from the Keto version and others may benefit more from the regular version of DHEA.

Kontak Spray Nasal P+B: Same as Super Good Stuff Nasal Wash.

L-Carnitine: Helps turn fat into energy. Taken in the morning. My hope was that it would help with energy. I cannot say if it helped or not.

L-Lysine: Goal was to reduce viral load. Not sure if it helped or not.

LL-37: Peptide that actually kills pathogens. Hope is to help reduce pathogen loads. I feel like it has helped slowly over time.

L-Phenylalanine: Amino acid to increase production of cate-cholamines/neurotransmitters for focus. It would ramp me up too much, and then I would wear myself out, making it a net negative.

L-Tryptophan: Amino acid to help boost serotonin and feel better and help with sleep. I thought I noticed a subtle effect, but long-term use was not effective.

Lauricidin: Same thing as monolaurin. Antiviral, to help reduce viral loads, which would increase energy and overall well-being. I still take this, and this helps. When certain viruses were flaring up, I would double my dose, and it would help me feel better.

Liquid Vitamin D3 with K2: Vitamin D3 is critical to mental health, immune system. I get my levels tested regularly and keep it in a good range. Even if I walk in the sun every day I still have to supplement with quite a bit of vitamin D. I can't say I felt notice-able effects or can pinpoint it to vitamin D, but I know keeping it in range is vital for my Lyme recovery.

Lomatium: I took this for antiviral, to help reduce EBV (Epstein-Barr Virus). I am not sure if it helped.

Lypo-Spheric Vitamin C: Same effects as Vitamin C Buffered Salts Powder.

Magnesium Oil: I spray this on my legs at night. Helps with magnesium depletion, which is common with Lyme. I feel it helps me sleep deeper.

MegaSporeBiotic: Probiotic that is supposed to be able to survive the stomach acid and be stored at room temperature. I have taken this off and on pretty much my entire Lyme journey, and it has been critical in my recovery and my gut health.

Methyl B-Complex with Methyl B12: B vitamins to help overall health. I took methyl forms because I have genetic issues with the MTHFR gene. I know it helped, but a doctor later told me I shouldn't have been taking the methyl forms.

Methyl-Guard Plus (Thorne): Large amounts of methyl form of B vitamins. It gave me plenty of B vitamins, but the methyl forms could have been too much for my body to handle and may have made it harder for me to get better.

Milk Thistle: Same effects as Seeking Health Liver Nutrients.

Mora: Antimicrobial to help kill off Lyme and other coinfections. Same experience as with Houttuynia.

Multi Mineral: Minerals to help with deficiencies often caused by Lyme. Common nutritional deficiencies are things like copper, zinc, magnesium, and iodine. I can't say for sure how much this has helped.

MycoPhyto: Blend of different mushroom extracts that was supposed to help modulate the immune system, so that my immune system wouldn't overreact and wouldn't cause too much inflammation, therefore making me feel better. This may have actually made me worse.

NAC: Supposed to increase glutathione levels and help detox the liver and kidneys. Goal was to help me overall get better. Not sure if it helped or not, but I think it might have.

NAD: Supposed to restore neurologic function, reduce aging, and improve mental clarity. Goal was to help heal the body over-all. I noticed improvements using NAD, especially in the short term. Can't say whether it was completely critical to my getting better or not, however.

NAT Ketones: Ketones were supposed to help me stay in a keto-sis state, which would lower inflammation and make me heal from Lyme. This did not help me in my Lyme journey.

NeuroFlam (Apex): Goal was to help with brain health by reducing oxidative stress and lowering inflammation. Not sure if it helped or not.

Oil of Oregano: Supposed to help kill off parasites and Lyme bacteria. Not sure if it helped or not, but it definitely is very strong and was rough on my stomach.

Olive Leaf Extract: Supposed to help with acute and chronic virus infections. I am not sure if this helped or not.

Oregon Grape: I took this when my test results were coming back saying I had high strep count, which was making me feel bad. I started taking it in hopes it would lower the strep. I am not sure if it did or not.

Pantothenic Acid: One of the B vitamins necessary for fatty acid metabolism. Lab work showed I was deficient in this, so I took it for a while. I am not sure if it helped or improved my situation, just that I needed it.

Para-Gard: Supposed to kill off parasites with ingredients like wormwood. Pretty intense ingredients. It was a bit rough on my stomach. Not sure whether it caused any improvement or not.

Plum Balls: Supposed to help with herxing, reducing symptoms when they were flaring up hard. I have no idea if they worked or not, but they definitely tasted good.

Pregnenolone (MIH Brand): Taking this because I have a deficiency in it, according to lab work. This is to help my mental clarity, mood, and healing. I feel like it has positive effects.

Probiotics (Various): Gut health is everything. Probiotics not only have made it so I didn't collapse from antibiotic use, they also have played a critical role in my Lyme journey. They have made a big difference, and it wouldn't have been possible to get better at all without them. I have cycled different probiotics my entire Lyme journey and still do.

Psyllium Husk Powder: Taken every morning to help my gut, bowels, colon, etc. move along and stabilize blood sugar. I believe it has helped me feel better in the mornings. I no longer take this due to hearing that it has high lead content.

Red Root: Helps with detox. Supposed to help remove dead cells from the lymphatic system. Can't say 100 percent if it has helped, but again, the overall combination of all the tinctures I have taken together has helped me get better.

Regular B-Complex (Unmethylated): Same as the B-complex above but the non-methyl forms to make sure I am not over-methylating. It is supposed to improve overall healing and energy. I believe it has helped.

RepairVite (Apex): Goal was to help heal the intestinal tract and intestinal lining. Can't say one way or the other if it helped or not.

Resvero (Apex): Delivers resveratrol, which is support to help your cells. I cannot say whether or not this worked.

Saccharomyces Boulardii: Taken to help push bad yeast and mold toxins out of my gut. I cannot say I felt an immediate effect, but I know this is helping me overcome the mold toxicity that I have.

Samento, aka Cat's Claw (NutraMedix): Goal is to help the immune system, help with inflammation, increase white blood cell count. I know this has helped me because I noticed different effects at different dosages, and a couple times I would run out and forget to reorder and then see a dip in my overall state when I wasn't taking it. My doctor would have me up my dose when I was experiencing bad herx reactions or not feeling good.

Seeking Health Liver Nutrients: My blood work showed elevated liver enzymes, which was indicative of poor liver health. I took this combined with Milk Thistle while placing a castor oil pack every night on my liver. After three months my liver test results became healthy again.

Selenium-Iodide: I was deficient in these nutrients according to lab work, so I am taking this supplement to help bring it back in order. Iodine helps with thyroid, which is essential to feeling better. I can't say 100 percent this helped, but it probably has.

Sermorelin: I injected this every other night. Supposed to help with natural production of growth hormone, to help heal the body. I cannot say if it has helped me or not.

Serrepeptase: Supposed to help break down the biofilm, like the biocidin. Not sure if it helped.

Se-Zyme Forte: This is a selenium supplement. I was probably deficient in selenium, so this would help with mood and immune function. Not sure if it helped or not.

Sida Acuta: Herbal tincture to help kill off Babesia, a coinfection that acts similar to malaria. I would notice herxing and increased negative effects when taking this tincture (meaning pathogens were dying and were releasing toxins into my body), so it was doing something.

Stevia Drops: Studies showed that stevia helped kill off Lyme, so I took stevia drops based on that. I don't know if stevia drops even have the same effect as stevia powder, and it is not well documented that it helps. I have no idea if this helped or not.

Super Enzymes (NOW): Digestive enzymes to help process food. This helped reduce some of the symptoms when eating. I still take digestive enzymes with each meal.

Super Good Stuff Nasal Wash: I had a staph infection, and my nose was red. I took this to help reduce the staph infection after finishing a round of a medication I was spraying in my nose. It helped get rid of the redness.

Teasel (NutraMedix): Supposed to help kill Lyme and relieve pain and chronic fatigue. I took it with so many other tinctures it is hard to say for sure, but I feel like it has helped me.

Thiamax: Mold toxicity interferes with the body's ability to use thiamin, which can cause depression and low energy. The body needs thiamin and magnesium to function properly. This is supposed to be a better-absorbed form of thiamin. Definitely helping me feel better as part of the mold protocol.

Thymosin Alpha-1: A peptide to boost immune function, similar to Thymosin Beta-4 in my current protocol; this has helped me a lot.

Thymosin Beta-4: Intended to increase Th1/Treg and reduce Th2/Th17, along with providing additional rejuvenating properties. Goal was to help shift the immune system to more intracellular action to get at the Lyme, since Lyme hides in the body. This has helped me a lot.

Turmeric: Goal is to lower inflammation, which will help with healing and feeling much better. I can't say for sure if turmeric supplements help or not.

Turmero (Apex): Help support the immune system and liver's detoxification. Can't say if it helped or not, but I still take turmeric supplements in other forms. I would still take this if I needed it.

Ultima Replenisher Electrolytes: Taking electrolytes to help make sure I stay hydrated. This has helped me, and I still take when needed. Sometimes I would notice an immediate improvement in mood when taking this.

UltraVir-X: Contains astragalus and other ingredients to help with immune support and inflammation. No idea if it helped.

Viobin-Prometol: Fortified wheat germ oil concentrate. Rich in vitamin E, policosanols, and essential fatty acids such as linoleic acid. Goal is to help balance fatty acids for overall improvement of my cells and body. However, it contains gluten, so I immediately stopped taking it after realizing that, since gluten is bad for me.

Vital Nutrients Glycine Powder: Was supposed to help me sleep deeper. Made my sleep worse, and I felt like shit in the morning after. Stopped taking it.

Vitamin C Buffered Salts Powder: High-dose vitamin C is supposed to have antimicrobial effects and support the immune system. I hoped that it would improve my situation overall. I know it has helped because when I did high-dose vitamin C IVs I got relief. I take vitamin C as a supplement in powder and liquid form every day.

Vitamin Code Multivitamin for Men (Garden of Life): A multivitamin I took for a while to have a general intake of vitamins and minerals since my gut health is not very good, which would lead to malabsorption. I would say taking a multivitamin throughout the Lyme journey is very important and has helped me a lot.

Vitamin D3 + K2 Softgel & Liquid Dropper: I was low in vitamin D when testing, so this is one of the supplements I take to keep it in range. Proper vitamin D range is essential for your immune system and feeling good overall. I test this every now and then to make sure I keep it at a high-enough level (but not too high).

Yerba Prima Daily Fiber Caps: Supposed to help stabilize blood sugar to maintain stable energy levels and keep my body stable throughout the day. This helped me wake up and go to sleep with better blood glucose scores.

WHAT I'M TAKING AS OF JANUARY 2022— ALTHOUGH I DO NOT RECOMMEND TAKING THIS MANY SUPPLEMENTS ANYMORE AND I HAVE DRASTICALLY CUT DOWN

Medications

- Testosterone—0.25 mL 2x/week (200 mg/ml)

- Liothyronine—5 mcg 1x/day

- NP Thyroid—30 mg 2x/day

- Anastrozole—1 mg tablet 3x/week

Supplements

- CBD+CBN at night (when needed)

- Magnesium Oil Spray

- L-Lysine—1,000 mg 1x morning, 1x night

- 7-Keto DHEA—50 mg 1x morning

- DGL before meals (sometimes)

- Selenium + Iodine

- NOW Super Enzymes—1 capsule before meals

- Nordic Naturals ProOmega 2000—3 softgels/day

- Quercetin—500 mg 1x morning

- Garden of Life: Vitamin Code Men—1 cap/day

- Seeking Health: B Complex Plus Methyl-Free—1 cap/day

- Swanson Turmeric—1 cap/day

- Hawaiian Astaxanthin BioAstin—12 mg, 1 cap/day

- Seeking Health: Liver Nutrients—1 cap/day

- Thorne Zinc Picolinate—30 mg, 1 cap/day

- Apex Energetics: Glutathione Recycler—2 caps/morning

- Apex Energetics: EnteroVite—2 caps 2x/day

- Gaia Herbs: Milk Thistle—2 caps/night

- Liposomal Glutathione—1 squirt/morning

- Liposomal Vitamin C—1 squirt 2x/day

- Apex Energetics Resvero—1x morning and night

- Apex Energetics Turmero—1x morning and night

- Saccharomyces Boulardii—1 cap/night

- Immune Power Immuno-Synbiotic—1 cap/morning

- Vitamin D3+K2 Softgel—1 per morning

- Nusava D3 K2 Omega 3 MCT Oil

- MegaSporeBiotic—1 cap/day

- Prescript-Assist—1 cap/day

- Organic Psyllium Husk Powder—1 scoop/day

- Thorne Amino Complex—1 scoop/day

Daily Smoothie

- Frozen Veggie Ice Cube (homemade with a food processor; mix of random vegetables)

- Udo's Oil 369 Blend

- Barlean's Forti-Flax

- Garden of Life Raw Organic Perfect Food Green Superfood

- Vital Proteins Original Collagen Peptides

- Moringa Powder

- Phosphatidylcholine

- Hyperbiotic Prebiotic Powder

- Chicken Isolate Protein—1 scoop

- Apex Energetics ClearVite-GLB—1 scoop

- Japanese Knotweed Powder

- Organic Chia Seed

Tinctures

- Samento—2x/day

- Burbur Pinella—10 drops 2x/day

- Oregon Grape—1x/day

- Red Root—2x/day

- Cordyceps—1 drop 1x/day

- Cilantro—10 drops 2x/day

- Teasel—10 drops 2x/day

Peptides/Injections

- Sermorelin every other night—0.15 mL

- NAD+—0.5 mL Monday/Wednesday/Friday

- BPC-157—0.3 mL 5 days on, 2 days off, 4 weeks on, 1 week off

- Thymosin Alpha-1—0.3 mL 5 days on, 2 days off, 4 weeks on, 1 week off

- Thymosin Beta-4—0.3 mL 5 days on, 2 days off, 4 weeks on, 1 week off

- LL-37—0.15 mL every day

Other Practices

- Parasite Cleanse Supplements during full moon (see below)

- I microdose mushrooms when needed (before sales meetings if tired)

Histamine Supplements

- **Histamine Digest, Quercetin 300, Perimine**: These three supplements have helped me with eating food. I used to have reactions almost every time I ate; now my reactions are not as severe. My reactions had to do with Mast Cell Activation.

- **Pepcid, Claritin**: While taking these two supplements at night I have noticed I sleep a lot deeper. I wake up in a deep sleep where I don't know what is going on. That never happened before. I was always waking up too early or sleeping very lightly. I stopped taking them recently to prevent the risk of them having a rebound effect later.

Binders

- **Activated Charcoal, Medi-Clay, Chlorella**: Binders to bind up the mold toxicity, so I can detox them out of my body.

Anti-Parasite Supplements

Para 1, Para 2, Para 3, CandiBactin-AR, BioToxin Binder, ZeoBind: These are all supplements from CellCore Biosciences. I used to take these once a month around the full moon because that is supposedly when parasites come out. It is a whole protocol with antiparasitic ingredients and binders to bind up the dead parasites. I started this due to multiple people saying that parasites can inhibit progress in getting better from Lyme and that clearing parasites can make it so you can eat more foods. I have noticed feeling better once the six-day cleanses are over. Also, near the end of one cleanse and while doing a colonic, the nurse practitioner believed I passed a tapeworm!

ABOUT THE AUTHOR

TAYLOR "TJ" NELSON has battled Lyme disease since 2016 with remarkable success. Although it initially robbed him of everything and he is still improving to this day, he has entrepreneurship in his blood and just won't quit, managing both the Lyme condition and learning how to succeed despite his health issues. He continues to work relentlessly to improve his health while growing his multimillion-dollar company, Direct Solar. Contact him at TJ@WalkTheLyme.com.